Awakening the Divine Feminine:

18 Stories of Healing, Inspiration, and Empowerment

Compiled by Laura J Cornell, PhD

Awakening the Divine Feminine:
18 Stories of Healing, Inspiration, and Empowerment

Divine Feminine Yoga LLC
100 Sedona Street
Sedona, Arizona 86351

First Edition
ISBN: 978-1-7333923-2-7
First printing June, 2021

Library of Congress Control Number: 2021910153

The content of this book is for general instruction only. Each person's physical, emotional, and spiritual condition is unique. The instruction in this book is not intended to replace or interrupt the reader's relationship with a physician or other mental health professional. Please consult your doctor for matters pertaining to your specific health.

Cover Design by: Expert Insights
Layout Design by: Expert Insights
Editors: Expert Insights, Laura J Cornell, Hyla Hitchcox, Anne Ondrey, and the entire team of Co-Authors

Dedication

To the women of this planet —
thank you for reading
these stories and sharing our journey.

To our sisters, mothers, grandmothers, aunts and
daughters in the celestial realms —
We see you.
We feel you.

Thank you for your presence in our midst.

Introduction

Never before has the Divine Feminine been so needed on our planet. The ecological balance of our climate is precariously disrupted. Species extinction accelerates from our own human folly. Isolation, loneliness, and mental illness are increasing, while political divisions and polarization continue to deepen. The conflict and anguish over our COVID year, still not behind us, have only deepened human isolation and the disparity between wealthy and poor nations, wealthy and poor people.

Unending war propagated by the military-industrial complex is also not behind us. Military spending continues to increase and covert groups seek new threats with which to scare humanity. The threat of an alien invasion or of "other" (code for non-United States) nations beating us in the "race" to militarize space is currently ramping up. This is only one in an unending string of false threats intended to convince the population to accept crippling military spending rather than funding human happiness, human thriving, and abundance for all.

The Dalai Lama's now-famous phrase, "The world will be saved by the Western Woman," is truer now than ever.

As women, we hold in our bodies the power to give birth, and we care ferociously for what we give birth to. Women are the tenders and the carers, and our emotions are naturally primed to attune us to the needs of others. We hear the cry of Mother Earth in her suffering, and we desperately want to stop it.

Mother Earth's suffering will stop only when humanity as a whole — both women AND men — collectively raise our consciousness to the level of love. We need to become an ethical species of the cosmos, resolving to use our technology only for good. But we are not there yet, and time is short.

Women awakening to the Divine Feminine force within us is a powerful medicine for our planet. This is the medicine we need today — the medicine of love, wisdom, and truth.

The Divine Feminine is already awake, already whole and perfect. But we must rouse ourselves from the slumber in which we have forgotten Her. We can open to Her, letting Her flow through every channel in our body, then share Her with our families, friends, lovers, students, and clients.

Awakening is a collective project. Together we weave the fabric of our wholeness. Our stories reveal our individual truths: who we are, what we offer to the world, and what we most long for. Through each other's stories, we feel empathy. We experience each other as mirrors, reflecting back to us our whole and perfect selves.

Telling a story is an act of generosity. The collection of stories you hold in your hand represent the heartfelt gifts of these women as they harvest the wisdom of their lives, sharing what they have learned from facing challenges with courage and humility, authenticity and integrity.

This book contains stories of women who transformed their most profound difficulties into a source of strength that they now use to help others heal. These women allowed themselves to believe that their stories — no matter how mundane, shocking, or painful — are worth telling, and in fact, realize that it would be a disservice to the world *not* to tell their stories.

How do women learn about the power of the feminine? Through living our lives, through loving, being sexual, having babies (or not), raising children, being wounded, healing, grieving, teaching, and through practicing tenderness and strength.

Read this book and the stories it contains. Then bring your powerful self forward. Bring your own story to the circle.

Bring your love, your peace, and your passion. You are needed as a woman at this time. Your voice is needed. We invite you to join us.

Laura J Cornell, PhD (*Yogeshwari*)
Sedona, Arizona, May 20, 2021

Table Of Contents

INTEGRATION

SACRED FEMININE HEALING

FULLY HUMAN — FULLY DIVINE

WOMB WISDOM

Chapter 1
Birthing the Wild Feminine Within
Through Miscarriage, Adoption, and Childbirth

Esther Wyss-Flamm

Body take me deep
Down into the knowing
Of the mothers who walked before me.
That I may sit at their feet,
Listen to the ancient tales,
Taste the broth of their bones
Cupped in the sacred palms of this earth.

— Prayer I wrote after a miscarriage

Dedication
For the Beloved Spirit Children that reside within us, some birthed into this World and some remaining in the Spirit Realm: their fierce determination fills me with awe and certainty that I am not alone. For the steadfast loving presence of Bradley, my life partner. This story of my awakening to the age-old wild feminine inside of me would not be what it is without him.

* * * * *

The primal desire to be a mother is not something I ever thought I'd have to fight for. And yet, that is exactly what I did over the course of seven years, with a determination and fierceness I never knew I had. The stories we weave come from the scars on our body, the tightness in our breath, the slur in our voice as we speak of heartbreak, breathtaking joy, and discovery residing in the core of our being. This story comes from that place.

Growing up, I stalked the stacks at libraries, a voracious reader of myths, fairy tales and sagas. I loved climbing trees, running across open fields, and listening to music in a cluttered basement with Maggie who lived next door. At night, I lay sprawled out on the driveway leaning into the warmth of our dog and stared up at the stars.

I had dreams that landed me in intricate plots featuring freakish monsters and magical forces that protected me. I vividly remember one of them took me underground into hollows among the roots below, to find a cave guarded by an elder woman stirring a giant cauldron of bone soup over the fire. She ladled some of the simmering soup into a bowl and handed it to me. I ran away. The ancient wild feminine was terrifying; decades would pass before I could make peace with this part of me.

Over time, I started to walk past the climbing trees with low-hanging branches; Maggie went away to boarding school; and I forgot to gaze at the stars. I was preoccupied by homework, by wanting to "be normal," and later by a career with social change organizations. Starting with the U.S. Peace Corps, this work took me (and a few years later my partner Bradley and me), to far-flung places overseas. The horizon in front of me felt wide open and exciting.

Which brings me to the moment when I was sitting in the cracked pink bathtub of our home in Lusaka, Zambia where Bradley and I were living at the time.

I lay surrounded by soothing warm water, precious water. Drought was a factor at that time in Southern Africa. It felt indulgent to draw a warm bath that afternoon. I watched a thread of red blood flow out between my legs – the dark color blending into the clear water in wisps and swirls, as life blood met Life Element Water. Tears streamed down my cheeks, as I lay in the tub in the sweet embrace of warm water on skin, knowing that I would release the kernel of life that had died deep inside of me. Tears turned to sobs, my eyes gazing up at the branch of the guava tree outside as it knocked against the window.

All I could do is release and let go into the moment. And the moment meant that the pregnancy I had held for three and a half months was now sliding out of me. I knew the sadness was real: the joy and secret feelings of wanting to hold a sweet baby that I'd carried in my body dissolved here in this moment of blood meeting water. My back was aching, my cramping was intense, I felt vulnerable and scared.

That's when I heard words in a voice that I didn't yet know coming up inside, a female voice, telling me: "Listen to your body; it knows what is coming. You are not alone. Trust that your body knows what it needs. This is a time to let go." And here I was, with a soft, clean cloth beside me, letting gravity do what needed to happen. I felt her voice, and then her presence guiding me, telling me to breathe just a moment longer. This was what I had fought hard to deny for days, keeping my legs tightly wound together, ignoring the bloody streaks that had appeared on my underwear, making light of the fluttering cramps.

She went on to tell me: "Stand up, Esther, it's time to stand up." I stood, and a clump of blood and tissue slid out of my body into the palm of my hand. I placed it on the soft cloth. Later I wrapped up the cloth and put it into a small box that I placed under the bed.

In the coming days, my sadness quickly turned into anger and frustration. I told myself that it was time to move on and get rid of the box. Once again, that reassuring, serene voice returned to bring me the deeper clarity I needed: the box was to stay where it sat under the bed.

I lay despondent. Only I knew it was there, the little box of a dream interrupted. While I was aware of what had happened clinically, another part of me sought deeper understanding in fleeting images appearing in dreams.

A few days later, I sensed her letting me know it was time. I buried the box by the giant elephant ear leaves under the guava tree. This felt real and right. I was able to stand up again, and felt strength surging up inside. I was able to reconnect with Bradley, able to face the world around me.

Still, unfriendly thoughts developed in my mind: how could I have messed up this most fundamental part of being born female? A deep mistrust of my body, a sense of having been failed began to settle in. These perceptions were reinforced by comments from family and friends. "Miscarriage has never happened in our family before" and "all I have to do is touch my husband's underwear and I end up with a baby nine months later."

It was at that time that I noticed the power of sitting in stillness. When I sat quietly at the beginning of a day, even for just ten minutes, I could breathe freely. I observed that those judgmental thoughts weren't real, that they were fabrications of my mind. Then I felt better in my body and could move on with my day.

Life flowed back into its rhythm, I dove deeper into my job, and the voice that had guided me through these difficult months receded into the background. Yet, the work was no longer as satisfying. A year later, Bradley and I decided not to renew our contracts and began graduate studies in the midwestern United States. In a few months, I was pregnant again. Yes, I told myself, the stars are aligned this time and I'll become a mom.

It didn't happen. The ultrasound at twelve weeks indicated there was no heartbeat. I was told that the pregnancy was not viable and that it would be easiest to get a D&C. One moment I had a small orb of light and hope inside, the next I was empty, the pregnancy vacuumed out of my body in a sterile hospital setting. I never saw it, never felt it flow out of me; no one could see, it was just me and my invisible loss.

Throughout this time, the voice I had heard guiding me stayed disconcertingly quiet and I didn't have a box to bury.

The confusion of pregnancy loss became an obsession, and I noticed how easy it was to stay and wallow there. I was typically either worried about what I needed to do to get pregnant and keep a pregnancy or thinking about what I needed to do to distract myself and move on with the rest of my life. I landed on entitled feelings that "I'd paid my dues," and then followed up with self-reproach. Or I'd brush off the experience with, "Oh well, no big deal. It wasn't meant to be. Don't dwell on it. Just move on." Try again.

More cycles of miscarriage followed, punctuated by myriad tests for both of us, hormone injections, and a slippery slope of increasingly invasive interventions.

I hated the waiting room of the high-risk OB/GYN practice, walls plastered with baby pictures and heart-shaped thank you cards. The doctor had a stellar reputation; he wore cowboy boots as he strutted from room to room filled with clients yearning for full-term pregnancies. For me, the process would run its course. After trying for months, I find out I'm pregnant, go in for an ultrasound, learn there was no heartbeat, submit to another D&C, and then try again.

That summer I caught a glimpse of myself in the mirror of the lavatory of an airplane on our way to a family reunion, giving myself a carefully timed hormone injection. I saw a steely-eyed, thirty-something-year-old woman, and barely recognized her. The drone of the airplane vibrated my body. I took a deep breath, and felt a deeper, softer knowing take hold inside. Relief flooded through me as her voice returned to tell me, "This is not your path."

I was tired of trying to force something, playing games with my body and tricking my mind.

In the months after I jumped off the fertility roller-coaster, I listened more closely to her voice. I noticed my connection to her strengthen during that early morning meditation. My regular yoga practice also allowed me to get past the noise to discern something deeper within me, something that reminded me that all was already and always okay. The kind and gentle voice that occasionally rose to the surface during these times made it okay to dissolve into tears and feel my sadness.

Bradley and I wondered about the instinct-driven need for our genetic material to be part of a new life we'd bring into the world. Was this rooted in a desire to see my face in that of my child? In the end, the need for a biological connection didn't seem as important as wanting to parent a child. We decided to pursue adoption.

And we soon landed on a whole new mess of questions: Adopt locally? Nationally? Internationally? Interracially? We pursued an open domestic adoption, and a few months later were selected by a teenage couple to become parents to the interracial baby they were expecting. I picked up the call minutes after the baby was born, a girl, and we headed to the hospital. Long-held tension released in my shoulders as I held this tiny bundle. Finally!

And then we found out about a rare genetic condition that the birth mom carried, tuberous sclerosis. Tests revealed that the baby was born blind with lesions in her eyes and other organs, lesions that would develop into invasive tumors covering her body including her vital organs. We were told she would not live long; that she would never be able to live independently.

I wanted to believe this child was meant to be ours. Medical professionals and social workers pulled me aside, asked me to reconsider and imagine what caring for her would mean for us. We pulled back and let go of this baby; predictably, a new layer of guilt and shame dropped onto my body. As I struggled through this time, I could feel the now familiar voice console me, help me pray for this sweet baby, and hold me through the grief that followed.

We waited. Another adoption fell through when a grandmother showed up to parent the newborn baby boy.

The social worker urged us to consider international adoption, and after another nine months, a photo arrived from Vietnam: a tiny girl named Thinh, wearing a frilly dress looking up at the camera. She needed parents. I felt something rise up inside of me as I gazed at the photo. Hope does spring eternal! We said yes, and we sat, and we waited.

Thinh's adoption papers made their way through layers of bureaucratic review one slow step at a time. We waited past her first birthday, her first steps, her hospitalization with pneumonia, her move to a foster family, her entry into full-fledged toddlerdom. Six months later, we were notified we had less than a week to travel to Da Nang, Vietnam, to meet this little girl. On the wings of this promise, we expedited tickets and visas, endured sleepless nights at the hotel, and showed up early at the gates of the Children's Center. We were handed a little wisp of a girl. Thinh looked as exhausted as we were. She struggled and cried when I tried to hold her. Bradley had more success; she allowed him to rock her to sleep in his arms.

The following day we officially became Thinh's parents in Da Nang's city hall. After another week of jumping through administrative hoops, the adoption was sanctioned by the U.S. Embassy in Ho Chi Minh City. We fell in love with this spunky tiny toddler who ran away wherever we went, already set on taking off on her own. We named her Maya and flew back home as a family.

In the adoption community, there is much talk about the strength and resilience of love residing at the heart of this arrangement. But flying from the vibrant life we found in Vietnam to the stark midwestern winter, I felt heavy with the truth. Intercultural adoption meant that we were tearing Maya from her homeland, her context, the language she was just learning to speak.

None of us adoptive parents like to think too much about this side of the arrangement. We may work hard to build bridges with our child's culture of origin (honoring celebrations, cooking the food, and building relationships with a nearby Vietnamese community), but in truth, we chose a path our privilege and resources allowed us to take, and didn't look much past the tunnel vision of our deep desire to be parents. Who is to say that I would be the right mom for this sweet bouncy toddler? How can we ever know? We trust, we love, we take it day by day, we believe and hold on to each other.

Many times over the years, I've had to surrender and let go into this truth and trust the guidance of the gentle, wise voice within me. Uncertainty has been a powerful teacher on this parenting journey.

As a couple, the ease of our lives slipped away as we transformed into becoming Maya's parents. Our connection as a threesome became strong and steady. Those first weeks turned into months, and then a move to family student housing in California. Amid as diverse a community as one could possibly find, Maya grew and thrived. I remember her as exuberant, a girl skipping with her Mom, riding on the bike with her Dad, commandeering monkey bars at playgrounds and digging enthusiastically in our community garden, sleeping heavily after a story at the end of each day.

We agreed that Maya needed a sibling. We had sent in an application to adopt a second child when I discovered I was pregnant. Sigh. I knew this path all too well. I felt a protective wall go up inside. I knew my body would again contend with cells coming together to form another being.

This time, the knowing voice inside of me reminded me I needed to be present for Maya and the strong, determined energy she was bringing into our lives.

My body embraced the pregnancy during those first weeks, and the ultrasound let us know there was a heartbeat.

"That doesn't mean anything," is what I said to Bradley.

"We've been here before."

"Let's not think about it," he said.

By the way, asking a woman not to think about a baby growing inside her is like asking her to cut off her head – not possible.

My body started growing like the squash on the vines of the community garden outside. We cancelled our plans to adopt a second time. Maya became enthralled by "her" baby that would be arriving. Could I contradict her? No, I couldn't; it was her baby. As I pushed her "higher, Mama, higher!" in her favorite swing, I knew I would not be carrying a pregnancy to term without her vibrant presence in my life.

I felt myself release into the experience of growing a baby. The seventh month brought me a most exquisite and unexpected gift. I was visited by a dream of the Spirit Children. I saw four children running toward me on the horizon, waving. At first, I didn't know who they were, but then I recognized them as the Ones who didn't find their way into the world through me. They came close enough for me to see their smiling eyes. In West Africa, an area of the world I'd lived in for seven years, there is a word for Spirit Children: 'abiku,' which means "those who are elsewhere waiting to be born." I woke up from this dream, feeling relieved and happy that they were nearby, so beautiful and fine.

Our son Theo was born in natural childbirth with a woman named Luna as the attending midwife. At one point, she guided my hand to touch his crowning head between my legs, a fleeting moment of grace, followed by sensing him slide out of my body and then gently placed on my belly. I drew him into my arms, an awkward bundle covered with tissue and streaks of blood, squinting eyes and a mouth that soon found its way to my breast.

*****

I can't know what would have happened had I not had that first miscarriage or the courage years later to adopt a child.

I do know there is no such thing as willing a child into the world – each is bestowed on us to be their guardian for a few years, and then this time passes.

This is a story, my story, about learning to claim my whole self. I moved from a promising career with exciting travel, immersion in different cultures, privilege, status, recognition, and a good income, to find myself in a bathtub bleeding as I lost my first pregnancy. At the time, I thought adding children to my life would flow seamlessly. It didn't.

Instead, I woke up to a primal part of me that sought connection and renewal. My body drew me into a deeply personal journey of transformation. Learning to listen for and access the wild feminine within taught me to surrender to the rhythms of life and death, to drop into stillness, to move and loosen the parts of me conditioned to be cerebral, driven, and goal-oriented. I can now draw on the fierce energy of the feminine to move more freely, ride waves of creativity, and savor the short time I have on this planet.

My former self stands in awe and surprise at how I find myself now: a light worker and mind-body healer. I support women stuck at a crossroads on their path and guide them to reclaim their own vitality and gifts, often in the thick of everyday family and working life.

As I work with my clients, I draw on my wealth of experience and academic training while rooted in a foundation of inner strength and body wisdom I was unable to access before.

I write this knowing there are many women who choose not to parent a child, who instead hold cherished Spirit Children in their hearts that are dreams for themselves, too often deferred. So many of us have literally or figuratively experienced miscarriage and are trying to heal parts of our lives that feel blocked. This is a tall order when we are conditioned to strive, excel, and seek certainty in a fast-paced world defined by change.

And yet, sooner or later, we all stumble upon events in our lives that become opportunities to dive into deeper knowing, to experience our innate wisdom, wholeness, and connection. The ancient feminine is always there, beckoning. When we begin to listen, events that appear to be setbacks turn into perfect, unexpected set-ups for the next stage of our lives. Eventually, we find ourselves able to sit fearlessly with this wild, wise part of ourselves, and drink from that bowl of bone soup offered to us.

I close with an invitation for you, dear reader: What moments come to mind when you've sensed an opportunity to step into your deeper wisdom self? What might you need to release to allow the wild feminine to rise up and have space to roam in your life?

About Esther Wyss-Flamm, PhD, E-RYT

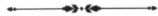

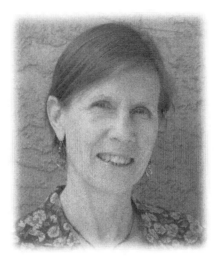

Inspired by her own and her clients' experiences with the wild feminine, Esther is a healing guide, a mindfulness coach and yoga instructor. Her passion is mentoring women to reclaim their innate vitality, to thrive, and live joyfully into their life purpose. Whether one-on-one or with groups, she adapts and personalizes mind-body practices that reduce anxiety, give voice to dreams, and clarify next steps.

Esther worked for over a decade with women's leadership education and community health organizations in the U.S. and overseas before completing a PhD in Organizational Behavior. She is the owner of White Flame Yoga in Philadelphia and serves on the board of several community-based organizations. Esther begins each day with gratitude.

estherwyssflamm.com
Owner & Lead Instructor, White Flame Yoga:
whiteflameyoga.com
e-mail: esther@whiteflameyoga.com

Chapter 2
Reclaiming the Female Body
Through Abortion

Jen Antill

I squat above the toilet and pee on the pregnancy stick. It's a toilet in a public bathroom, luckily a single stall. These four tin walls around me offer some semblance of privacy from the winding line of strangers standing outside of it, waiting to relieve themselves. I set the pregnancy stick lightly down on the sink. Now, I wait. I feel kind of numb. Like I'm living someone else's life, almost hovering above myself in this bathroom, detached and floating. I peer down at the white stick on the sink. It's a plus sign. Apparently, that means I'm pregnant.

Everything feels like "apparently". Apparently, I now have to deal with being pregnant. Apparently, now I have to make decisions. *Apparently* is something being done to me, something outside of my control, something that demands me to move closer to it and breathe into its face. I feel like a teenager, frustrated and disgruntled that I now have to deal with the reality of my situation. Can't I just continue backpacking and traveling throughout New Zealand? Apparently, I have to make a decision that some women may be required to make in their lifetime. Apparently, I'm old enough to be a woman.

The last couple of months make sense now. My breasts have been sore. From what I can remember, I haven't had a period in about two months. I had to pull over on the side of the road to throw up a couple of weeks ago. But it didn't even occur to me. I *can't* be pregnant. I can't be pregnant because it would mean I've ruined the expected, perfect trajectory of my life. Being pregnant means I'm either going to become a mother at the age of twenty-three or have an abortion and neither option will be considered flattering by my parents or the fundamentalist Christian community I was raised in.

David, my boyfriend, and I go to the nearest medical clinic in Auckland. I get a blood test that reveals the seriousness of my pregnancy. Now it's official. The nurse smiles at me and congratulates me but I don't smile back. She gives me a purple balloon to carry out of the clinic as a symbol of celebration. I'm about eight weeks along and rapidly growing.

David thinks we are ready to have a baby together. He's excited, hopeful for our future. He wants me to keep it. He wants to raise our baby in the sun and soil and teach it how to grow eggplants, tomatoes and squash.

David and I have been together a year and a half — the longest relationship I've had so far. Months before we got to New Zealand, David asked me to marry him and gave me a ring that had two doves twisted around it — a ring he found at a gas station outside of Blythe, California. I tentatively agreed to the proposal — mostly because marriage is an intoxicating fantasy for me, a nice daydream, but when it comes to the reality of it, I'm scared of making choices.

Making choices reminds me of the closeness of death. There are certain choices we make that we cannot undo. They stay with us for our entire lives. They are irreversible — a tattoo on our soul. I don't feel ready to make these kinds of decisions. I still want the feeling of a blank slate. I want the feeling of perfection. The reality of love and relationship is often too messy and too imperfect.

David decides that he cannot accompany me back to the States — he cannot bear the idea that I may not want to keep our baby. I'm relieved. I would never be able to make this choice with his heavy preferences hanging over me. I would first want to make sure I was pleasing him, rather than facing his imminent disappointment in me for not being ready to become a mother.

Back in the States, the first abortion clinic I go to is in the same medical building I used to go to as a child. I've taken this elevator thousands of times. I've smelled the antiseptic in the hallways and rubbed my arms to try and keep warm in the cold air-conditioning on many occasions. I know this office. But I'm here for a different reason now.

As I check in to the office, a nurse with a thick German accent sets me on a scale and takes down my weight — 145 pounds. She tells me how having children was the worst decision she ever made. She was not happy as a mother. She felt her children held her back from the things she really wanted to do. She tells me how she thinks I am making the right choice.

As I step off the scale, I start to cry. I think it might be a light cry, one that I can easily hide. But my face starts to twist, the sides of my mouth start to cave and I cannot hide this wail. The wail that emerges from me shakes my whole body.

The wail takes over and soon I am sobbing and shuddering — my whole body shaking. The wail is now the *thing* in the room — it has a presence and energy of its own. I cry for the German nurse who didn't want to be a mother. I cry because I feel alone. I cry because, in this moment, I need softness and tenderness and there is none to be found here.

I cry because I feel the enormity of this decision. I cry because I'm afraid I am making the wrong choice. I cry because I'm weary and scared. I cry because David is not here and ultimately, I know I can't rely on him — our relationship will never last. There will come a time when I will have to grieve its ending. Maybe I'm already grieving it now.

Because the wail is so loud and persistent, the doctor tells me he won't perform the procedure on me. I have to wait out the weekend and come back on Monday. When he tells me this, I resist and protest. I try and wipe away the tears, telling him I'm ready — he can do it now. I will pull myself together. I'll stop crying, I promise. But he shakes his head, no, not today. I feel powerless. I feel defeated. I cannot change his mind.

I step out into the parking lot and I finally feel *it*. I feel my clarity. I feel my knowing. I feel my sureness. The anger led me right here to this spot. As soon as my choice was taken away from me, as soon as the doctor told me "no", I knew what I must do. I *cannot* have this baby. I *will not* have this baby. There is something that happens in my body — it feels like a metal rod that wraps itself around my spine and roots itself into the ground. I am sure. This is clarity. I will not have this baby. I feel ferocious. I feel rage. I feel an unrelenting desire to discontinue something. I no longer feel unsure. I no longer vacillate. This is not a decision I make.

My body makes it for me. My body tells me about the steel rod inside my spine. It tells me of all the qualities of a steel rod — unbending and unmoving — something that never disintegrates.

I make another appointment for Monday, this time at a different clinic. On Monday morning, my father and my two best friends accompany me to the clinic. They shield me as we walk through the abortion protestors at the entrance of the clinic. I feel a little bit like a celebrity — I'm doing something important.

Once we are inside the clinic, there are certain places that no one can go with me. I have to go alone into the examination room where they give me another Ultrasound to confirm my pregnancy. I slip into the gown; I take the Valium and the cervical dilator and I know there is no turning back. Once the cervix dilates, this baby won't be able to grow. It will be the end. There is a second waiting room that I'm taken into and now, I'm not alone. There are six other gowned women and we are all taking the cervical dilators and Valium. We hold small, white Dixie cups in our pale hands. We are not turning back. We are going forward. The

Valium helps us walk forward as if there were a little mist around us — sometimes it's hard to walk forward when you can see everything so clearly.

As I lie down on the table in the dark operating room, the nurse tells me it will take five minutes. It's a very simple procedure. I hold her hand and there is scraping. She tells me not to breathe so fast or I will pass out. There is pinching and scraping. I have no idea why there is pinching and scraping. I don't know what there is to pinch or to scrape. I have no idea what my insides look like and these particular insides feel important to know about — more important than the insides of my intestines or liver. With these particular insides, the ones they are poking and scraping, I have to be careful. Without knowing it, I created something that could one day live and breathe — all on its own. These are the kinds of insides you have to come to know. These are the insides I cannot stand to ignore any longer.

They can scrape and poke and prod me on this table. They can tie me, cut me, and singe me. I am at their mercy. I am the biggest devotee of this surgical world in this moment. I need them. I can't live without them. I am in their temple.

Without them, I become a mother. I don't like depending on people I don't know. I don't like the feeling of being at someone else's mercy. I don't like the feeling of giving over my fate to anonymous gloved hands. There is too much at stake here. These things of blood and life and motherhood — I have left them on the table for someone else to tend to.

In this moment, I promise myself that I will never leave it up to someone else again to tend to what is mine.

As a woman, there are certain things that are mine to hold — to be the sacred keeper of. There are certain things that I have ownership and rulership over. These things must be protected at all costs. If I do not recognize these very specific things that I have ownership over as a woman, if I do not hunt my power and swallow it whole, then I lose it all together. In this moment, I promise myself that I will never feel this powerless or clueless again about the things that are mine to keep sacred and to hold. I'm embarrassed and ashamed. I have not been a knowledge keeper of this body of mine. I'm guilty of ignorance.

I realize that my body will always win. It will always bring me back to the physical world. My body ultimately has the say, it has the final word. Pregnant. Sick. Alive. Tired. My body is the Queen — she rules all. Without her consent, I do nothing. I bow to my Queen in this moment and promise to serve her with my entire heart. Never again will I pretend that another ruler has the throne.

The promise I make to myself is to learn about my body. I want to learn everything I can. I want to shine a light into the darkness of the caverns where there was scraping and pinching. I want to understand how one moment I was pregnant and the next moment I was not. I want to understand how *I* can be the hands that dictate my future.

It takes me a couple of months to recuperate and rest after the abortion. I journal. I cry. I write letters to my baby who was never born. I name her *Mara*, a name that comes to me in a dream. The name *Mara* holds many meanings in many different languages. But I look to the ancestral roots in my bloodline — the Irish and Swedish meanings of the word.

Mara is the word for sea in the Irish language and in Swedish, *Mara* means nightmare. Perhaps Mara was never meant to be physically embodied, but to be returned to the eternal sea, the grand unconscious, collective constellation of souls. In my prayers, I encourage her to try and come into this world again, through a more willing vessel.

A couple of months after the abortion, I go and visit David who is now in Thailand. I still love David, even though I felt unsupported and betrayed by him throughout the process of the abortion. But it's hard for me to let go. I don't want to face my own grief and so I entertain the fantasy of him and

I still creating a life together. While we are in Thailand, I get the name "Mara" tattooed on the arch of my left foot but half of it washes away as I walk in the ocean moments after getting it done. The name remains on my foot — half legible and half invisible.

The last night I see David, he comes inside of me without warning. Without a condom, without birth control and without trying to pull out — he stays inside of me, limp and lazy, denying what he's just done. This is perhaps the deepest betrayal of all. Not only does David not accept the abortion or honor my decision but he blatantly disrespects it and rejects it. I know after this; I will never see David again. This is the experience that I needed to finally let go. This is the unforgivable moment. Again, the steel rod comes — the anger, the clarity.

After I get back from Thailand, a new chapter of my life starts to call me. I am free. Free of David. Free of motherhood. I have time to search for and gestate the knowledge I am hungry for. I don't want to waste this time. I feel like it's been generously handed back to me with the condition to use it wisely. I want to become the woman I have been running from — I want to become a woman who *knows*.

The following month, I find myself on a living room floor in Asheville, North Carolina. The living room floor is covered with purple and gold pillows, while the incense burns in a holder on a nearby bookcase. The blue ridge mountains hold me and I feel their strength around me, cradling me, inviting me to safety. Before me, stands a woman with wild grey hair and thick, metal spiral-shaped earrings. She is well-spoken like a magical poet. She is telling me, along with ten other women, a story about how women naturally give birth — how when a woman is left undisturbed, she does not lie on her back, working against gravity in order to push her baby out. Instead, she kneels or squats or finds another position that allows her body to work with gravity and that allows her baby to be caught with her own hands. Once she has birthed her baby, she lays her baby on the floor. She does not pick her baby up. She leaves her baby undisturbed. She takes a moment for herself. This is *her* moment — she claims her motherhood, she claims her power. She will only later claim her baby when she is ready. The tears stream down my face as I listen. I cannot look away. I will *never* look away. My prey — the access to this knowledge that has been denied to me — is finally clenched between my jaws. This is the birthright of all women, to know secrets like this whispered to us on living room floors.

I went on to study with this wild and magical teacher for one year. Through her teaching and guidance, I became a midwife. I hunted and claimed the knowledge that rightfully belongs to all of us as women. I then apprenticed with a midwife in Santa Fe, New Mexico for one year, witnessing multiple forms of birth from home births to hospital births to water births to relatively unassisted births. I learned how to help women administer herbal abortions, taught women about their menstrual cycles and how to naturally conceive.

I became an expert in the field of women's health where I had once been blind. To this day, one of the most powerful and profound experiences I know of is to sit on the floor with women and illuminate the secrets of our bodies — helping one another find our way to the knowledge that is our birthright.

Today, I offer myself not as a birth midwife, but as a Midwife of the Soul. The more I worked with birthing women, the more I realized I wanted to reach them before they became mothers. I wanted to reach deep into ancestral lines and lineages and work with profound energetic and emotional patterns. I wanted to help stop the generational passing down of pain, trauma, and hurt. Today, I work as an Astrological Counselor and Midwife of the Soul to women all over the world. As women, the healing we do impacts our legacy and our children. It impacts the generations to come. With our knowledge, with our healing, we weave the future webs of our world.

About Jen Antill

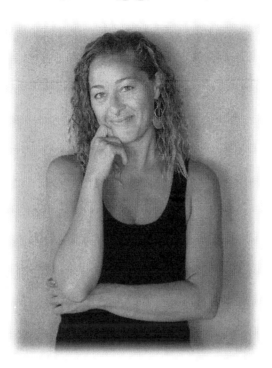

Jen works as an Alchemical Astrologer and Counselor to women all over the world — guiding them to find their truth, clarity, and power.

Jen lives in Sedona, Arizona with her partner, Heathar and their dog Alice. You find out all about Jen at www.jenantill.com and follow Jen on Instagram @jen_antill_astrology.

STRENGTH

Chapter 3
Healing My Broken Back Through the Divine Gift of Yoga

➡➤•◀⬅

Deah Jenkins

Some people say they can't do yoga. They feel like they have to push hard to assume the shape of a pose or to look a certain way in a pose. That's why I share my story.

In my times of injury, my yoga hasn't looked the same as other people's yoga. Much of it has been simply visualizing the movements along with breathing. What can change everything is being open to healing, being open to receiving, and exploring whatever range of motion is available to you in each moment.

For me, yoga is the day-to-day experience of living. I lead a course that helps students bounce back from burnout. While determination is an important element, self-care is equally critical.

Everyone can apply everyday self-care elements of yoga somewhere in their life, in a relationship or at a job. It's the art of living well. We all have that capacity within us if we shift our perception inward.

This is the story of several defining moments in my life, moments that made me who I am. All of my life has led me to yoga, to healing. My life hasn't been easy, but it has been an amazing journey.

I was the oldest child of 3 siblings. At age 11, when I was both a tomboy and a daddy's girl, my mom moved my two younger siblings and I out of the state — overnight and without explanation. I hadn't even imagined my parents getting divorced. But now I was in a strange new place without my dad or my friends. I took on many responsibilities due to my mom's increased work schedule. I babysat and made meals for my ten-year old sister and four-year old brother. No more fishing with my dad. My days were full of adult activities.

However, when I was on my own, I became an adventurous teenager who loved the great outdoors. We had a reservoir and a swimming hole that I frequented with my friends outside our small Mississippi town.

On one particular early summer day when I was 15, I sported a brand-new, black bikini. I was even happier that my first boyfriend, who I had broken up with, showed up at the swimming hole. We were having a bit of a happy reunion when we climbed up a ladder to the high point where we'd grab a bar on a rope swing to jump out and drop into the water.

On one attempt, he and I were grabbing the bar together. I was thinking more about him and my new bathing suit than our stability on the bar.

I was the only girl who'd ever swung on this rope swing and I had always been able to do it. But on this swing, I let go of the rope at the wrong time. I remember the fall in dreamy, slow motion. I felt a thud that shuddered through my body, which was followed by a bump and then another series of bumps.

I don't know exactly what happened next except I know my friends were holding my head out of the pond with the rest of my body spread out in the shallow water. I couldn't feel my legs. I couldn't move.

There were no cell phones in those days and someone had to drive to the nearest pay phone to call an ambulance. It seemed to take forever but the rescue crew finally came. The medics strapped me to a backboard and drove me to the nearest hospital 30 minutes away.

I remember imploring the hospital staff, "...please don't cut it!" as they snipped off my brand new bathing suit. I was given a shot, I'm assuming for pain, and I became violently nauseous and started vomiting. They flipped me over, to keep me from choking, so now I was upside down and vomiting.

In that moment, I felt a change, a shift. I don't know if it was my body's innate wisdom or Divine intervention or both, but it was surely a miracle.

It started with my breath. I went into my breath and a state of calm came over me that I now know intimately from years of yoga and meditation. A shower of grace washed over me. For that, I am forever grateful.

From this place of peace, I became my own advocate. I let the staff know that I would not take any more medication.

This was a declaration of my sovereignty over my body and my healing process.

I was speaking up for myself. The way they would have treated me — the normal path — was not the path for me. I didn't have resources or people to guide me on whatever my path was. The longer I was there and even though I was in pain, I knew with great certainty that I wasn't going to follow the medication path.

Once I was in my hospital bed, I spent a lot of time alone. My mom was busy and unavailable. She had remarried and had another child who was only two years old, plus my other siblings. She was only able to visit me once in the hospital during the weeks that I was there. Many years later she didn't even remember that I'd broken my leg as well as my back in the accident.

My dad was an alcoholic. I now know he was heartbroken over the divorce. He lived several states away and was no longer a part of our life. I longed for my dad when I was in the hospital. I felt sure that if he knew what had happened to me that he would come and visit me. But he never did.

Since I'd had to grow up so fast following the move and the divorce, I was already self-reliant. As I lay in the hospital bed, I knew I was on my own. My teenage memory of that time is of feeling completely alone. I don't remember hospital staff coming in and out of my room. It was just me.

So I continued entering into that state of calm, meditating before I even knew what meditation was. I sensed I was being held and protected. I received peace, comfort and stillness.

I'm not sure how, but I knew to just breathe, to just be there. I knew I couldn't be anywhere else, and that my situation just was what it was. So I allowed it. I knew I couldn't change it. I couldn't make anything happen or make anyone do things for me.

I slid into that space where there were no thoughts, just breath and peace beyond understanding. I believe that's when I received the Divine gift of yoga. I didn't know much about yoga yet, but through grace, I was already living it.

The doctors weren't sure when or whether I'd walk again, or if I'd be permanently paralyzed. Even though I had no sensation in my feet, I visualized moving them. My recovery process moved inward and became deeply intuitive, as I connected with my breath and with visualizing movement.

Soon my healing sped up dramatically and I was improving faster than the doctors expected. I began to stretch and feel into the little bit of the mobility that I had.

I didn't have any explanation for what I was experiencing. Growing up in a small town in Mississippi, I would have called it answered prayer. I was simply being present and I felt calm. I felt relaxed. I had faith. I had a vision that this was *not* where I was staying — paralyzed and hospitalized.

I was determined to make a different choice. "I'm getting out of this bed. I'm going to do everything I can to heal. I'm going to be here, right now. There's nowhere else I can be."

It turned out my right leg was broken and I started to feel pain in my leg. What utter excitement to feel my legs — even if it was through pain! My aunt was a nurse at a different hospital that was a distance from the hospital where I'd been taken. She talked the doctors into releasing me early into her care. However, once I was released and arrived home, I was on my own with my siblings. There was no physical therapy in our town at that time and no resources. Healing was up to me.

I trained my younger brother and sister to take care of me. I had them pull me around the house on a sheet to get me where I needed to go. The phone, in those days, was up on the wall and as a teenager, getting to it was one of my first priorities.

After a few weeks, my aunt took me to a doctor's appointment where they removed the cast from my leg. The doctor wanted to recast my leg. I refused and was given a pair of crutches and returned home.

When I was a cheerleader at school, we stretched before our practice. I used some of those stretches to help regain my mobility. The accident happened at the beginning of the summer, but I recovered enough by fall to return to school, moving with some caution.

During my next defining moment, my capacity for resilience was tested again. I married and became a young mother in my 18th year. I labored without medicine, riding the waves of contractions and exhaustion.

My daughter, Jennifer, was born a healthy, big bundle of love weighing nine pounds and 21 inches long. Fortunately, she was a happy, easygoing baby who mostly slept through the night. I felt so much joy, bliss, and amazing love. I now had another passion: creating opportunity for her and nurturing her to adulthood.

My vision of mothering my daughter involved being home with her. But after losing one house and with the landlord threatening to evict us from a second, I had another defining moment: I went into business for myself.

I knew I couldn't let my daughter suffer from constant moves based on my husband's income. So I became a property manager. Through the years, I've learned to pretty much take apart and put together everything and anything — from washing machines to faucets to heating and cooling systems.

Even with my new business, I always kept my hand in holistic practices — picking herbs for tea or growing and eating vegetables. I signed up for a yoga class at my local YMCA.

Fast forward to a second accident in my 30s. While I was driving, my Jeep was hit by a semi-trailer truck carrying sod. I injured my right leg and developed searing sciatic nerve pain. Using the skills I'd developed, I kept going to my yoga class, positioning myself in the back of the room. I was only able to do about 10 percent of the class but just as I did in the hospital with the last accident, I visualized whatever movements I couldn't do. I knew it was working because it reduced my pain. If I missed class, my pain became worse.

I returned to that space of breathing and visualizing. A desire was growing in me to know how yoga worked, and why it worked so well. Despite some reservations about yoga based on my childhood religious beliefs, I filled out the training application. The day I sent it in, I went to my regular class and the fitness director at the YMCA asked me if I could substitute teach the class that day.

"Why me?" I asked. "Because you're always here and the teacher is not." This confirmed that I was on my path.

Once I completed my teacher training, yoga class after yoga class fell into my lap. I even started teaching yoga at my church where the members knew and trusted me, after years of my volunteering and participating in mission trips.

Any hesitancy I had felt about yoga based on my religious beliefs vanished and I felt sure sharing the practice was a wellness benefit for everyone.

During my recovery from the car accident, I was given a prescription for a massage. I didn't want to go. I thought massages were a luxury activity. I tried it and didn't like it that much. I couldn't relax. Still, I tried it once more after I'd been to a yoga class. I was amazed at how I could relax this time and how my body responded with suppleness to the therapist's touch after yoga. I began to realize that through yoga, I had the capacity to open my mind and allow my body to receive the benefits of massage.

Secretly, I had always dreamed of turning my fascination with the body into a career as a doctor. But at this point, I decided to change my focus. I decided to become a massage therapist. This led to decades of training as a personal trainer, a cranial sacral therapist, a reflexologist, a clinical herbalist and a medical aromatherapist.

I love doing bodywork. I love being part of other people's healing journey. I love seeing how it offers them an opportunity to go to that inward place where they can direct their own healing. I love hearing, "After your massage, I slept eight hours for the first time in a week," as a client told me recently.

I try to help clients reveal their own inner power: to breathe and connect. This superpower within each of us is available when we become present to ourselves and to our environment, just as I did when I was in the hospital.

My continued studies have confirmed the enduring truth of what entered my life with that first awareness of the breath in the hospital. At age 15, the path that emerged before my eyes unfolded in a way that I couldn't have imagined in my wildest dreams.

A wonderful blessing for me was seeing my daughter graduate from college. This defining life moment is perhaps my favorite other than her birth.

It was a sunny day in the North Carolina Black Mountains, the highest mountain range in the Eastern United States. Jennifer's dog and best friend, Rusty, broke away from where we were sitting and crossed the stage with her as she received her diploma!

My daughter is an independent, self-assured woman. She's an organic farmer, a beekeeper, and a jewelry designer. Seeing her grow into her own woman with free expression has been unmitigated bliss. It's helped me enter into the love of a mother's heart, which I've been able to share with others, including my dad, after he had his own spiritual journey recovering from alcoholism. I sat by him and held his hand as he passed from this earth.

My dad was there for my first breath, and I was there for his last.

I believe all the years of attending my daughter's swim meets and leading her Girl Scout troops, listening to her and to her teammates and friends, prepared me for the work I do now as a health and performance coach.

Many of my clients are high achievers. They're dynamic leaders and teachers, caring and giving it all they've got, pouring themselves into their work until they're depleted. They find themselves feeling unsure and sometimes unable to relax and to rest.

I help them to focus on finding their breath, moving their bodies, being present with accepting what is and visualizing their truth: all the same skills that have formed my path.

Lately, I've been working with high performance athletes. I remind golfers to remain in the present, and not to worry about the previous shot. I ask them to couple their awareness to their breath, to focus with clarity, and to use visualization. If you find yourself distracted by someone or something, just come back to the breath. Be present with the sensation of your hands on the club. See the ball and the direction you want it to go. This helps them win, which after all, is their goal.

When the COVID pandemic started in 2020, I developed a remote program called Embodied Resilience. Students hadn't been open to remote learning before, but now, stuck at home, they were open to this new platform. For the first time, I was able to explore teaching online and it's been wonderful. Students have had a bit more time during the pandemic to allow the practices to make an impact in their lives and they've gained skills to help with immunity, lung capacity, stress release and high anxiety.

It's heartwarming to see how one class I lead — they call themselves "The Yoga Gang" — came together to support each other. One of the ladies' husbands had a hemorrhage, and everyone signed up to bring the couple meals and to get groceries for them. Yoga provided a connection and a sense of giving towards each other within the group.

These students are doing what is called Karma yoga, which is being of service and it's an important part of the practice. It has a cyclical element to it. You offer to others and somehow this generosity ends up coming back to you. The more I teach, the more I experience that benefit. It returns to me and from me to my students in the ebb and flow of giving and receiving.

Yoga takes effort but that doesn't mean it's unpleasant. It does require patience and continued work as well as taking a hard look at our habits.

"Our yoga is really just our routine in life, our daily moments," I tell my students. "It's each moment. It's the breath."

I am so inspired to see yoga work for my students, to see their own wisdom revealed and how it carries them forward.

Often, we need to implement these tools of yoga again and again, year after year. I've recently suffered yet another car accident and I am recovering from a traumatic brain injury.

I continue to apply the tools: breathe, connect, visualize, and relax.

I believe I was given this gift. The only way I can describe what happened in the hospital that day is that I experienced grace, freely given. It created my purpose in life. It drives me. It's always felt like I had no other choice. Discovering, learning, and now teaching these tools is my life's work, but honestly it doesn't feel like work. It feels like a natural evolution from one breath to the next.

Try these tools for yourself. See where you want to be on your own path. Believe it. Breathe it.

About Deah Jenkins, E-RYT, LMT

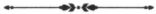

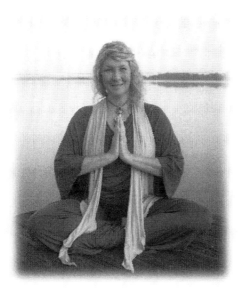

Deah Jenkins, E-RYT, LMT is a Mindful Performance Coach with an extensive background in holistic health and personal training. She is a licensed massage therapist with over 10,000 hours of practice, a certified Yoga Therapist, a Continuing Education Provider for Yoga Teachers, a clinical herbalist and a medical aromatherapist.

Deah loves helping her clients sleep better, decrease pain, and get back to enjoying their lives. She is especially proud of helping golfers win tournaments while reducing pain. Always an avid student, Deah is a doctoral candidate in Phytotherapy. She is an herbal educator who has an herbal apothecary where she creates a highly effective, individualized line of herbal pain reduction creams and sleep teas.

Visit Deah's website to experience "Meditation Made Easy," and check out her Vitality Restored Course and line of herbal creams and teas.

http://www.1LightWellness.com

Chapter 4
The Calm Within The Chaos of Special Needs Parenting

Jane Kleiman

As a kid, I often pretended I was a witch or a priestess or a queen. I had what I call my first spiritual experience sitting by the river near my home. I was in 8ᵗʰ grade. It was dusk. As I watched the lights move in and out of the trees in the hills across the water, time passed. I must have moved into some kind of meditative state, because once I "came to," I felt as though I had newly arrived in my own body – every one of my senses heightened. It felt like I had magic powers. Preternatural. It was an incredible feeling!

Though I tried to stay in touch with this part of myself, expectations of life and responsibility sent it to sit on the sidelines, only calling it into the game on rare occasions.

In my 30s, I shifted careers from video production to Massage Therapy. I was making ceramic art, had my own business, had a rich, daily yoga practice, and ample free time to have a full social life. I remember thinking: *This must be what a charmed life feels like* — doing what you love with ease.

That was before all the attempts to get pregnant, the infertility treatments, the tentative positive pregnancy results (*I'm happy to tell you, Ms. Kleiman that you are "mostly" pregnant.*), the difficult birth, the near impossible nursing (when I discovered what "listen to your gut" meant) and the seemingly innocuous pediatrician visit when the doctor suggested some early intervention (*I'm sure he'll catch up.*)

We then received the "Your Special Needs Child" packet in the mail, which led to a 20+ page evaluation of a severely developmentally disabled baby, countless hours of therapy, years on end of sleep deprivation (10 to be precise), glacially slow progress, marital strife (the divorce rate is 75% for couples with a disabled child), career loss, loss of self, loss of joy, and the arrival of my new state of being: hypervigilance. Eventually, we came to know what to expect, and by the time my son was about 7, we had arrived at what seemed like a semi-regular life. We'd finally found a rhythm, and our life was easier than it had been in a long time.

****

In 2012, when my son was 10, I saw that the Kripalu Center for Yoga and Health was offering their Yoga Teacher Training in New York City in a one-weekend-per-month format over the course of a year. I had loved Kripalu Yoga since my friend Nicki brought me to a class while I was visiting her in upstate NY. I gravitated toward Kripalu teachers whenever found them. When I first went back to a yoga class when my son was 2 years old, the teacher was a Kripalu teacher. I remember weeping at the end of class, feeling like I'd come home again. I'm still friends with her to this day. It was January. Training started in February. I enrolled.

I would spend the better part of the next year completing my training, one weekend at a time in New York City. It was glorious to spend lunch hour walking around the village where I'd lived for so many years. We began in the dark and gray of February in the Northeast and moved through the gradual awakening of the city to spring. As the city and earth sprang to life, I too was renewing.

The weekend format meant I had the whole next month to learn to integrate yoga into my life as it was now. That meant after-bedtime practice instead of a glass of wine. It meant using my breathing and awareness practices as I moved through my day, and when I was actually *in* my life not just when I was still or on my mat.

Spring turned to summer and the heat increased. I practiced in the pool while my son splashed in his happy place. As the sessions resumed in the magical place that is New York City in the autumn (yes, it's really like it is in the movies), I felt a calmness, a slowing down, a reserve of strength and emerging and power that I hadn't felt in what seemed like forever.

Fall quickly became early December, and it was time to plan for graduation weekend.

The arrangements for my son's care were a production. Skills from my former career kicked in to set up all the plans: the child care, the meal and medication instructions, transportation arrangements, share contact information across the long list of people involved. Do all this elaborate planning, and well, cross your fingers! You'll be fine. Your son will be fine. Oh, and by the way, your husband, the only person you've ever left your son with for more than a day? Yeah, he'll be across the country on a business trip. Turn it over to trust.

As the *Bhagavad Gita* (one of the seminal Hindu texts upon which Yoga is based) teaches: Perform the action and let go of the fruits of your labor.

Honestly, I knew everyone could handle executing the plans, but I was not so confident they could handle my son's behaviors. As he turned 11, he had become increasingly aggressive when stressed or upset. He would drop to the floor, hit, grab clothing, and pull hair. So, the emphasis needed to be on prevention; make sure he's never too hungry, change the subject, promise him something he loves for doing a good job.

****

And then, there I was, finally, at the Kripalu Center in the Berkshires of Massachusetts for graduation weekend of my 200-hour yoga teacher training.

It was the afternoon of the last full day. The Graduation ceremony would be the next morning. I was so delighted to be here at "The mothership," as our lead teacher called it, where I had come for retreats and renewals so many times.

But there was something that was still stuck. I couldn't quite let go into the experience, and I found myself grasping for the big feeling, the full emotional release that told me something was shifting. I felt annoyed that it was holding me back from connection, from being fully present. I chose to interpret it as natural anticipation and invited myself to let it be. We broke for dinner before our final evening session, and I headed back to my dorm room with joyful exhaustion looking forward to some delicious Kripalu food.

I checked my phone.

My mom had called... Three times.

The message she left was:

"I'm in the car with Mina and Jackson. The police are here. They are going to take Jackson to the hospital. He was pulling Mina's hair and my hair and kicking me. The police won't take him home, so I'm going to follow them. Call me back."

It was the phone call I was dreading. Everything stopped. My first instinct was to pack up and speed home. 3 1/2 hours. At night.

I called her back. My son was already gone. On his way to the hospital in a police car. She was about to follow.

"Call me when you get to the hospital," I told her. "Did you give him a snack? Did you offer him ice cream when he got home?" Did you? Did you! *Did you do all the things*?

My poor mother was traumatized and in pain. That hair pulling hurts like hell, especially when he gets right at the scalp. Multiple times. Her grandson just attacked her. I believe at that point in time, he was still laughing as he did it. So, not only did it hurt; it was also disturbing. All of a sudden, this usually sweet, happy boy was maniacally laughing as he grabbed at her, pulling her hair, and kicking.

"Don't let them give him anything," I told her. Immediately, I thought, *Who can I call?*

With my husband in Las Vegas, there was literally no point in upsetting him because there was less that he could do than me, and he was in the middle of work and needed to stay focused. My son needed a familiar face, besides my mom, who he could refocus on, and who could more easily redirect his attention. All our appropriately jovial friends were still on the way home from work.

So, on a Friday night, I called his teacher. She was absolutely <u>that</u> teacher. The one you remember your whole life, and she knew how to handle his behavior. It felt embarrassing and desperate and intrusive and presumptuous, but I did it anyway. I needed help. This dear woman, I'll call her Joanne, picked up the phone, and I didn't even ask what she was doing. I just launched into it, and would she go to the hospital and meet them there and make sure they didn't do anything like try to admit him to a psych ward or restrain him or drug him unnecessarily? She and her husband were on their way out to dinner, but without missing a beat, they turned around and headed to the hospital.

And there I sat, alone in my dorm room waiting to hear from someone that he had arrived at the hospital and he was safe and calm.

If I didn't finish the weekend at Kripalu, I would not graduate. I had no idea what accommodations could be made in the case of an emergency, but I very distinctly remember reading that because I knew it could happen. And now, here it was. Happening.

Joanne called me first. He was in a bed chatting them up like nothing had happened. Exhale #1.

I asked Joanne to put the nurse on. "Whatever you do, don't give him anything. He needs to eat. Can you please give him some food?"

My mother must've called me next.

"The nurse brought him a sandwich, and he is inhaling it."

Joanne: "They want to admit him. I will take care of it."

Here is where I'm grateful not only to the people who support our family with fierce conviction, but to my own inner wisdom that had me call just the right person. Joanne was able to advocate for my son that he did not need to be admitted. This was an autism meltdown that was now over, and he needed to get home to his familiar surroundings. She was not taking no for an answer. In fact, she sent my mom, the only one who could have consented to such a thing, home. She and her husband would wait for him to finish his second sandwich and bring him home. When he arrived, the army of people I had called were there to greet him, and I knew he was going to be okay. Exhale #2.

****

I went back to my final evening session before graduation the next day. I was shaking, hungry, exhausted, and spent.

Frozen and in shock, I was just instinctively putting one foot in front of the other. Propelling myself forward–no expectations, no real attachment to what had just occurred because I HAD to let that shit go.

It was time to leave behind the belief that this life of special needs parenting controlled every part of me, that no one could handle it but me, that my son couldn't handle it or work through his difficulties with anyone but me. We both needed freedom. We both needed agency. We both needed to learn to trust. I needed to accept help in really big, rich, deep full body, gracious ways. Without holding back, without holding onto the guilt. I needed to deserve that precious help, and let it envelop me like the bear hug that I needed.

We entered the room and were split into groups. In Kripalu yoga, there are three stages. Stage 1: You do yoga. "Will". Placing your body willfully into poses. Alignment, and physical sensation are key. Stage 2: You do yoga/yoga does you. "Will and Surrender". You are still using your will to move your body, but you can begin to sense the movement as energy, the energy as movement. Stage 3: Yoga does you. "Surrender".

Swami Kripalu would meditate for 10 to 12 hours per day, and his body would spontaneously move into different postures and shapes as an expression of that energy.

Meditation in Motion

This was the evening practice. We were to enter the circle that our group had formed, come into meditation and then let the energy move us, as we were witnessed by our yoga community. Our sangha.

You've got to be kidding. I already felt so tender, so raw and vulnerable, unsure if I could even make it through the session. How on earth was I going to be able to do this? But I knew there was no way out except through.

There's really no way to describe the feeling of sinking so deeply into yourself and letting your body move in whatever way it wants, letting out moans, crying, raging while people simply witness you. Normally, it would have been hard to let go of self-consciousness, but perhaps the incident at home forced me to a place that I wouldn't have reached on my own. That evening, I was delivered a gift and I accepted. I moved. I don't know how. I breathed into the pit of despair and longing and shame and grief. I sobbed and moaned and curled up into child's pose whispering, "Baby, baby," not even knowing for whom I was speaking. I simply let go. I gave it all up to "what is". I detached from the constant *struggle* and *conflict* and *aching* and *wanting things to be different* and *missing the person I was* and *hating so much of what was now my life*. I just gave in. And I was absolutely changed forever.

Being able to let go and trust is a key part of my story's origins and yet, I was absolutely married to the belief that this kind of surrender and trust only comes as a culmination of a dramatic experience — an intense deep retreat experience or a life-changing tragedy or crisis — not something you can just live in every day. I'm still working on the everyday part, but what I've come to understand and fully believe with all my being is that it doesn't have to be hard all the time.

****

I didn't do my teacher training because I had a burning desire to teach. I had a burning desire to stop yelling at my kids. To stop feeling so shitty all the time. After graduation, I taught some friends and discovered *I am a damn good yoga teacher.* However, I had zero interest in a job in a yoga studio, subbing until I could fill a class or teaching at 6am.

It was while I was sitting at bike camp that summer, that I understood who I wanted to serve. It was my second year hosting iCan Bike, a five-day camp to teach kids with disabilities to ride a two-wheel bike independently. As I sat in the bleachers with the parents watching their kids gain a skill that they had not been able to teach them on their own and weren't sure would ever come, knowing all too well the guilt they likely felt about that, tears would stream down our faces.

I realized that the joy I was connecting with was the parents' joy, and how rare and fleeting it can be. I realized I wanted to help other special needs parents have more of these moments. More moments of letting go of the guilt, of simply and only feeling the joy, and feeling the full and loving support of those around them. Maybe feeling like they, too, could take on something that they never thought they could do. It occurred to me that offering a yoga class specifically for them might help them to find that, as it did for me.

So, I founded *The Calm Within The Chaos*, a monthly yoga and support circle for parents of kids with disabilities. My initial tagline:

"If locking yourself in the bathroom with a glass of wine is your idea of relaxation… This circle is for you."

Turns out, there were quite a few of us in those locked bathrooms. We shared our stories. We moved and remembered what it's like to actually *feel* relaxed.

We used all of the tools of Kripalu Yoga. We sat in witness of each other in both the pain and the celebrations. We learned *how* to celebrate. We understood that we *deserved* to celebrate, and accept help, and be happy and fulfilled adults. It was a sacred space where we could come together so we could fall apart.

The year of the pandemic has re-introduced, reinforced the idea that we must learn to be where we are.

It has laid bare the parts of our lives that don't work. Many special needs moms have joked that we are probably the most prepared for this kind of life. Isolated, without social interaction, needing to let go of expectations and change entire ways of living at a moment's notice. Welcome to OUR world.

I've never stopped learning. With my son's school gratefully open, I have continued to support our parents while getting attuned to Level 2 Reiki, as well as learning about the nervous system, trauma response, and embodiment principles that can help us stay grounded and feel safe.

The more I can stay connected to my body and my senses and get my mind to sit down and take a break, the more I am able to *maintain a deep trust in myself.* The more I feel like I did that moment by the river when I knew something had happened but I didn't know what, and it didn't matter.

I've gotten back in touch with a witchy, magical part of myself that had really faded away, and that I assumed didn't belong in a responsible woman's life. Letting her out to play has been a completion of a cycle, and it's brought me home to myself and enhanced my other practices, such as yoga and art. I don't have time for a lot of *doing*. I need ways of *being* that work and that help. My whole practice these past 8 years has been about seeing moments of my everyday life as opportunities to practice. "Let it be easy," one of my teachers said to me recently. That's the heart of what I teach.

Our lives are hard enough. You deserve to be seen as your best friends see you. A badass. A rock star. A kickass, strong woman who has so much to bring to life and needs a shoulder to both stand and cry on.

It's been the honor of my life to guide and witness the women in our circles as they come home to themselves. As they start businesses, get back to the writing they love, get their degree, or move on from the circle to find their joy in other endeavors.

I'm so grateful to all my teachers, to Kripalu yoga, to Dreamscape Healing Arts, Divine Feminine Yoga, and to my own stubborn determination to know myself and to find out how and under what circumstances I am happy; what activities, visuals, sensations bring me joy? What feels like ease to me? What does my life look, feel, sound, and taste like when it is "right" for me? And how do I know?

Yoga gives me so much, so many tools to find that out – really all the tools. Reiki keeps me in the place of letting go and trusting.

Something is shifting, a new phase. I'm stepping into a new level of leadership that feels so much closer to who I thought I'd be as that witchy, magical kid sitting by the river, and I can only hear the self-doubt when the wind is blowing a certain direction.

Today, I am the mom of a 13-year-old daughter and a 19-year-old son with Autism and I/DD (Intellectual/ Developmental Disability). He is a sweet, happy, super social young man who loves rollercoasters, the full moon, fireworks, the beach, *The Hobbit* and Larry David. He can't read sentences or write, can type only his first name, and would walk into traffic if he wasn't with someone to stop him. He will need supervision and assistance his entire life. I love him and my daughter with my whole heart. My husband and I are still happily married.

About Jane Kleiman

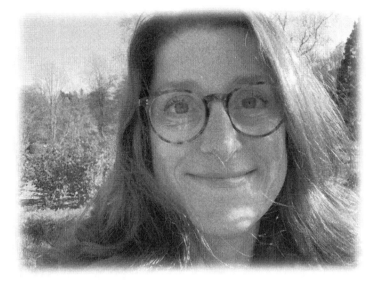

Jane Kleiman is a 200-Hour Certified Kripalu Yoga Instructor, Level 2 Reiki Practitioner, and lifelong spiritual seeker. In 2013, she founded The Calm Within The Chaos, A Movement and Support Circle for Parents of Kids with Disabilities, so that she could bring her experience, guidance and support to other struggling special needs parents.

She has also worked one-on-one with busy women who feel overwhelmed, stressed, and are longing to reclaim their lives for themselves. Her programs are in-person or online and will soon be developed into a guided at-home course.

To get information about future programs or to be notified of the launch of The Calm Within The Chaos At Home: https://www.thecalmwithinthechaos.com/join-our-online-community.html

Chapter 5
From Rejection to Resilience
A Journey of Love, Faith, and Yoga

Chona Villegas

People often say to me how giving and loving I am. I'm a kind person, a good person. I was a bedside nurse for 16 years and I've raised four happy kids, Czarina, Jonah, Zach and Isaiah. I own a yoga studio where I'm a friend and confidante for my students and co-teachers alike. I support my husband and together we remind each other to think positive, no matter what.

Very few people know my backstory, how I was raised, or how difficult my childhood was. I think it's important to understand because truly, it's a miracle that I'm alive at all, and that I'm able to smile, smile, and keep smiling.

When I was born in the Philippines, my mother was barely 18, unmarried, and did not finish high school. Her own mother had died when she was nine, and she didn't have a good relationship with her father, making her kind of like an orphan. She became pregnant with me by her neighbor—but they didn't have a relationship, so I was effectively born without a father. While my mother was in labor, she walked six miles, accompanied by an older woman, to the hospital where I was born. Imagine that! Walking six miles in labor the whole way.

Our community was not accepting of a child from a fatherless home with an unmarried mother. My mom and I were basically considered trash. We saw my father's family sometimes because they were our neighbors. I knew who he was, but he never acknowledged or even spoke to me. When I was seven, he married another woman and she was also hateful to me. My grandparents didn't even acknowledge me. In fact, my grandma used to spit at my mom and said unkind words to me when we passed by.

My mom was so young. She would just take off and leave me behind with her aunt who had raised her after her mom died. They did not have a good relationship. When I was young, they fought a lot: my mother, her siblings, and her aunt. Most of the time, growing up, I was with this aunt, who I called "Grandma."

My mom used to say she wished I was never born and tell me I was bad luck in her life. I'm sure life was hard for her, but when you hear those words as a child, they stick with you. Now that I am grown and a mother, I can look back with empathy for what she went through. It must have been very hard to raise a baby by herself with no education and so little family support.

At a young age and faced with so much rejection, I somehow found my own meditative way to cope. I have always been a very prayerful person. Even at that young age, I would just find a quiet space and pray. It was almost like yoga was already an inherent part of me. I don't know why. It was just who I was.

Growing up in a third-world country is so different than growing up here in the U.S. Being homeless here is probably still a better life than growing up in the Philippines, where I really had nothing. I endured hunger. I had to sell things just to survive. I was forced to grow up very quickly, learning life skills at a very early age. All I had was the community where I grew up and a few friends.

Despite the rejection and poverty, over time my faith strengthened. Somehow strangers would show up at the right time, helping me along the way as though the hand of the Divine had dropped them into my life.

Even though we were poor, my mom was determined to send me to a good school. You had to take a test to get into any good private school. My mom contacted an all-girls private Catholic High School when I was 12 and convinced them to let me take the test. I passed, but I had to work for the nuns as soon as I started there, since my mom could not afford the tuition.

Because of my social status, I had already experienced discrimination and bullying. At school, it continued. My classmates would say, "You don't belong here. You're poor! You're from the slums!" Most of the other students were from families that had money. Some even had drivers to pick them up from school. I had to walk to school with an empty stomach. I fainted many, many times at school because I didn't have food.

Meditation and my imagination helped me endure the bullying and the hunger. Many years later, talking to my husband, he said, "That was your coping skill, your survival skill." He was right. That is what helped me keep myself sane as a child.

My mom rented rooms in our house for supplemental income. The renters lived upstairs. We lived downstairs. When I was 14, one of my chores was to collect the rent at the end of the month.

One day, I went to get the rent from one of the renters. I had known this old man for a while. He was an ex-priest. My mom was so happy that there was an ex-priest living in our house because he would bless our house every day.

When I went to his room, he started touching my breasts and saying, "Oh, you've grown." Then he laid me on his bed, got on top of me and stuck his tongue inside my mouth. Thank goodness I had the brains to say, "This isn't right." I kicked him and ran away.

Though I got away from him, I didn't get the rent, so then I was afraid of my mom, too. I was spanked as a child if I didn't do things right. Fearful of being punished, I asked my friend to help me. I told her what had happened, and said, "You've got to go up there and get the rent." She did, and we never told anybody what he did. But it was impossible to avoid him.

It's hard to imagine, but there were about 20 people living in our house — all renters. We didn't have a stove. We didn't have any inside bathrooms, and we didn't have running water. There was just one common pipe that we could get water from. In the morning, everyone would line up to shower. We showered with our clothes on.

So, for almost two years, I had to face the old man every day when we lined up to shower. He didn't seem sorry for his behavior. It was very uncomfortable for me. When my mom praised him, it made me sick to my stomach. But I didn't want to tell anyone what he had done because it would be embarrassing for me and for my mom. Instead, I called upon my inner yoga, my survival instinct, to weather that difficult time.

When I was 16, we immigrated to the United States. My mom's sister brought us to California. We arrived in America on a Saturday, and my aunt took me to school on Monday. She didn't want me to fall behind, but I soon found out I was already behind. I encountered the same attitudes in the U.S. as in the Philippines — kids in high school were cruel. I didn't understand why there was so much bullying. No one was welcoming. Coming here in my teens and starting as a junior in high school was so hard. Those first two years were just plain torture.

I didn't understand how kids could be so cruel when I hadn't done anything to anyone. Even Filipino kids who were born in the U.S. constantly made fun of me. Somehow though, I didn't feel like I was a victim. I would look at them and think, "I feel bad for them because they're so stupid. They're so mean." It did not make sense to me why they would behave that way.

My survival skill carried me through. When things were really bad, I could just go inside and be in my own little world. I really have no idea how I learned to do that. I didn't know anything about yoga. But looking back, I feel like I've been mentally practicing yoga for my entire life.

In high school, I didn't want to be with any boys, especially Filipinos. I had the memory of the ex-priest back in the Philippines. Having gone to an all-girls school, I had not been around boys. Girls were forbidden to even talk to boys, so I really didn't know anything about them. I was very naïve. Plus, in our culture, your family background was very important. I was afraid if I dated a Filipino boy, his family would reject me because of my background.

My concern was based on my experience. I was very aware of why my mother wasn't married to my father. She didn't come from a good family. She was poor, with no mother or father. My father's family had money because his father was a politician. My mom was unacceptable to them.

Finally, in college, life improved. I was 18 and had my own apartment. My mom was out of the picture; she was like a teenager. I supported myself. I went to school full-time and worked full-time, which was very challenging. I had moved to Northern California to the San Francisco Bay Area and lived in Santa Clara. I ended up going into nursing school. During this time in college, I met some good friends who were Filipino immigrants like me, who spoke the same language, the same dialect. Then, when I was 20, I met my future husband.

He is Filipino, but he grew up in Canada. He was young when his family emigrated from the Philippines to Canada, and then when he was 20, his family moved to California. He was different from my other Filipino friends, like an outsider, because he didn't speak the language, although he tried.

We were just friends for the first 2 years. He was nice, but it was not love at first sight. I didn't look at him romantically at all, and he didn't look at me that way either. I wasn't interested in dating anyone then. I was very cautious. Plus, I really didn't even know how to like a boy. I couldn't picture being with someone because I didn't feel like I was worth it. Who would like me if they found out about my family? Thankfully, my worries were unfounded.

He was a fun guy and very smart. When we met, he was also a full-time student. He was broke because he was focused on school and would either not work or only work part-time. I was almost 22 when he finally became my boyfriend. My friends made fun of me. No money. Ugly car. They said, "What happened? Our requirement was a guy with a credit card and at least a nice car." His car was a Chevy Nova with a dent in front of the hood. When he turned the car on, he had to get out and hit that part of the hood so that the left side headlight would come on.

He was very nice and sometimes, since he had a car, he would offer my friends a ride. They would either refuse or they would accept a ride but try to hide. I used to tell them, "You know, I'm not dating the car. I'm dating the guy, and he's nice." That's all I cared about; he was a kind person.

When he got into UC Davis and I went to nursing school at Sacramento State, we began living together to help each other out financially. That was the only way I could finish nursing school because when you're in the program, you cannot work full-time. It would have been too hard for me to pay for the apartment, pay for my car, and go to college.

One beautiful and sunny summer morning, after a year of living together, we decided to get married!

Months before finishing my nursing program, we found out that I was pregnant with our first baby. At the same time, we got the exciting news that my husband was accepted into medical school in Washington, D. C. We lived there for four years and moved to Arizona for his medical residency.

My husband is now an interventional cardiologist. When our last child was born in 2006, I chose to stop working as a nurse. We decided, as a family, for me to be a full time stay-at-home mom to raise our four very active children.

I co-own a yoga studio now, but it was a long road getting here. My journey took me from the Philippines to the U.S., and Sacramento to Washington, D.C., nearly 3,000 miles from family on the West Coast, navigating many hardships along the way.

Nothing in life is easy. It's hard. Neither was opening my own yoga studio. When I first started it seven years ago, I did it by myself. I was going crazy. I didn't know what I was doing. I was not going to continue; then this woman came to me and offered to be a partner. I'd been praying for somebody. So now, I have a partner in my business, and for the last two years, things have been really good. Once again, the right person showed up at the right time.

Now, our studio is growing. Most people know opening a yoga studio is not going to make you rich, but it's a wonderful community. My niche is a little different than most yoga studios. It's not a young people's studio. It has become a circle of women devoted to helping each other. It's so nice to witness yoga changing lives, nourishing souls, and transforming my students and myself, mentally and physically.

When I first opened the studio, it was almost like a ministry. Random people would come in and just pour their hearts out. Whether they were going through divorce or various other hardships, they were drawn to the yoga studio. It's very strange how things just happen. Sometimes, as a studio owner, it's really hard, and then, when something like that happens, you feel, "Okay, there's a purpose for this."

The studio has become a very personal place in which people connect, share, and have become very close. I feel like yoga has given me a sense of purpose and a sense of self-worth.

Being a bedside nurse and being a yoga studio owner and instructor are both humbling professions. I believe nursing and yoga have very similar qualities. Both are about helping people. In life, we are in it together. My students come to the studio to take a pause and practice their yoga. Yoga gives them time to pause, breathe, and — I have a word for it — recalibrate.

That really is the essence of what I give to my students — a place and a moment in which to pause. Personally, yoga changed my life because I discovered that skill within myself when I was only a child and deepened it over time. There will always be ups and downs in life, but you can always take that pause.

I believe my yoga practice is connected to my faith. I have met my lifelong Christian friends through the studio and our love of yoga, sharing, studying and evolving together.

Recently, a nearby yoga studio closed, and one of the clients from that studio just happened to find my studio. She is a retired dental hygienist. She and her husband had moved to Arizona to start their retirement, but sadly, after just six months, her husband died of a sudden heart attack, leaving her a widow. She does not have children. She has a sister, who also doesn't have children, so her family is just the two of them.

When I first met her, she didn't have an open personality. Yoga was still very new to her, but before long, she shared with me that she liked it and she felt comfortable. I'm so thankful for that. When she first started, she would cry during practice. Although she was quiet and a closed person, I continued to encourage her to come to class and was supportive of her.

Over time, she opened up. Yoga has been a great therapy for her. She began to share her feelings about her grief with the larger group. It was so nice to see that, because at first she would only text me because I had told her, "If you need anything...let me know." So she did.

Now, almost two years later, she's a completely different person. Her practice is amazing. She really gets to the heart of yoga. She gave a glowing testimonial for our studio, saying it really changed her life and gave her something to look forward to. She has found a community. She has said she feels like she has found her second family. It has been so heartwarming to witness her transformation.

She is one of a group of 10 (and growing) women Yogis who formed a club during the pandemic when we had to close the studio. One of the other ladies lives nearby in a gated community that has a big park, and she invited us to offer a yoga class every day at the same time. That kept our practice going, while the studio was closed.

The women really bonded, and they formed a group they call Thirsty Thursday. They all love wine. Even though I don't drink alcohol, I enjoy joining them at their get-togethers.

Many of the people who come to my studio are new to yoga, so I keep it simple. I teach them what yoga is about from my heart.

When I introduce somebody to yoga, I always focus first on the breath. I encourage them to take their time. Most of us don't even think about our breathing. But with intention, breathing brings you to this very moment. If you can do that, that's your starting point of yoga. Then I begin to add some simple movement. I guess you'd call it moving meditation. That's how I introduce my students to yoga, gently and meditatively.

I have found yoga to be a powerful tool to have in life. Yoga is not just effective for your physical and mental health, but also for your soul. Life can be so, so hard, but yoga can help you strengthen your faith. For me, yoga and faith go hand in hand, and have been really helpful throughout my life, getting me through the toughest of times.

There will always be tough times. Even now, I'm going through a difficult house building process with obstacles at every turn. A lot of people at the studio know about it, and they say, "Chona, how are you still smiling?" I tell them, "Just breathe, right? Keep moving." It helps so much to focus on the positive instead of the negative, and just keep moving forward, so you don't get stuck in a rut. My husband is very good at reminding me to stay positive because he is very good at it. So, that is what we do — we keep our positive outlook, and we breathe together.

Life isn't easy. Sometimes, it's very, very hard. I often say to my kids and to my students: "It's okay not to be okay. Things will work out if you just allow the process to happen."

Just breathe. Embrace the pause. Within the pause lies the key to resilience. What was once the survival skill of an unwanted child has become profound teaching, shared by a gifted and resilient woman with so much love to share with the world.

About Chona Villegas

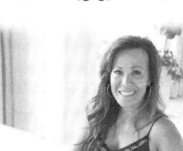

Chona Villegas is the founder/owner of Living Stone Yoga Studio. She has been practicing yoga since 2006. She completed the 500-hour Teacher Yoga Certification in June 2013 from the Southwest Institute of Healing and Arts.

Prior to life as yogini, she practiced a wide variety of nursing positions in a multitude of different disciplines. Her experience as a nurse combined with her passion for yoga allows Chona to provide a practice of yoga that focuses on alignment and structural integration.

Chona's classes are known for having a relaxing environment infused with moments of humor and real-life storytelling as they tie into her lessons. She provides practices in Hatha, Yin, Restorative, Wall Yoga and Yoga Nidra. In addition, she offers Stand Up Paddle (SUP) Yoga classes to private groups and those interested in exploring yoga in a fun or new way.

www.LivingStoneYoga.com

SURRENDER

Chapter 6
The Path to Healing for a Melanated Yogi

LaShanda Brown

I grew up an only child to a hard-working single mother with strong roots in the Black church. Like many other kids in my family, I spent Sunday mornings in Sunday school, and summers in church camp. My church upbringing shaped my worldview and instilled in me a desire to be of service to my community. Ultimately, this passion for service led me to a path of nursing and community service.

I stumbled upon yoga at my neighborhood YMCA during a time in my life when I was working twelve-hour night shifts at the hospital. I had been taking aerobics classes at the YMCA to relieve work-related stress, and one particular day, I happened to find a Black yoga teacher leading a class and felt compelled to join. Curiosity is what initially compelled me to give yoga a try, but the factor of representation had a strong influence. This new modality felt a lot more welcoming being offered by a familiar face.

From the very first class, what I discovered on that mat was a deep sense of peace and calm that I hadn't found anywhere else. That ignited a deeper curiosity to dive deeper into the world of yoga and meditation. I found more yoga classes and meditation classes outside of the YMCA environment, many of which were much more spiritual in nature.

The true turning point for me in my yoga journey happened in my first Bikram yoga class. I remember the intensity of walking into that hot yoga studio where the temperature and humidity are set to immediately induce sweating. Because the environment is so extreme, the instructors give very specific instructions on safety and self-care at the beginning of class. You would hear warnings to lie down when you feel lightheaded but DO NOT leave the room. I didn't like the idea of not having an option to leave; this warning made me want to leave the room immediately. But there was a clear method to the madness. Not only did I survive the heat, but I also came to respect the container that was set for our practice and trust in the teacher's ability to keep us safe.

Bikram yoga taught me the value of structure in life in the way the classes were always taught with the same repeating pose sequences. I learned in those classes that no matter how hard a task (or a pose) seems initially, it's always easier the second time around. I remember this as the first time I consciously began to translate survival skills learned on the mat to my everyday life. The structure of Bikram yoga helped me look for order and structure in work and home schedules, and value the wisdom that comes from leaning into predictable patterns in my world.

Bikram yoga had a format that I really needed at the time. In a regular yoga class, you try different poses and go through different sequences. You explore different poses as a way to get familiar with your body and how it functions best. You learn where you're strong and where you need additional support, and there's a lot of power in that knowledge.

With Bikram, you do pose number one twice, and you continue through a sequence of twenty-six poses without variation. You know exactly what to expect. When you hit that challenging pose that you absolutely hate, you know you've only got to do it two times, and then you get to move on. For me, that challenge was camel pose. It made me nauseated and light-headed, and that terrified me at first.

I quickly learned that this was how my body was responding to the shift in and out of this pose, and I learned to transition more slowly. While I still continued to have some nausea with this pose, I was mentally prepared for it and less afraid to tackle it during the class sequence.

Somehow that taught me about facing obstacles in my everyday life. The first time is always the hardest; by the time you do it the second time, you're over the dread. You're moving on to something else. That pattern became ingrained in my head. I wasn't afraid of something new because I knew that, even if a situation was new and difficult, it was only dreadful the first time. The second time I wouldn't be new at it anymore. I learned how to navigate it and I built the confidence to move past it.

Bikram was teaching me a different way to engage with life and its challenges that I've really come to appreciate. It's a very structured environment. I always knew exactly what to expect and I found comfort in that. It created safety and it built my confidence and strength a lot faster than the traditional yoga classes did.

At that time in my life, I was a wife, a mom to two young kids, and a nurse working twelve-hour night shifts. Working as a nurse, you meet people during the worst stages of their lives, and you bring home a lot of that—their stories, their pain and their traumas. Yoga was providing an outlet for me to process this secondary trauma that many healthcare professionals are subject to. Until then, I didn't have an outlet for my caregiver stress. I would work my shift, wash it all off at the end of the day, then return the next day and do it all over again.

One particularly challenging patient story that has always stuck with me was a man I had labelled as a 'frequent flyer.' He had a diagnosis of pancreatitis and would be hospitalized multiple times a year for severe pain. At the time, I could not process in my mind how genuine he was, and honestly thought maybe he was just seeking pain medication. He was angry, frustrated, and overwhelmed himself, and sometimes lashed out at the nursing staff. Of course, I offered him every ounce of compassion that I could, but I just could not connect to his struggle. And it's that feeling of helplessness that sticks with you as a nurse trying to provide care for someone that you feel you're barely making an impact on.

Helplessness is one sign of secondary trauma that nurses must navigate, that will surely lead to burnout if left unaddressed. I was learning to build resilience through the embodiment practices I was learning on the mat. At the point where I was edging towards burnout in my nursing career, I found yoga or maybe yoga found me. Yoga gave me a place to reset in a way that I couldn't find anywhere else.

Navigating a Health Crisis

While I was beginning to build a resilience practice that helped me with work-life balance, the true test came during my first major health crisis. In my early 30s, I began a four-year period where I was having severe abdominal pain and multiple visits to seek treatment, much like the patient that left such an impact on me. The doctors diagnosed me with gallstones that had created a cyst on my pancreas. This combination resulted in numerous doctors' appointments, emergency room visits, and hospital stays over the course of those four years.

In a two-year period, I had two major abdominal surgeries to correct the problems with my gallbladder and pancreas. Because of my pancreatitis flare-ups, it was pretty typical to be admitted to the hospital a few times in a year to be put on IV fluids and restricted from eating for up to 5 days so that my pancreas could rest and heal itself. And just to put things in perspective, I was still working full time in a hospital on night shifts, being a mom of two, and I was a full-time graduate student. To say those were challenging times would be a huge understatement.

In my follow-up appointment after my second surgery, I asked my surgeon what I could do to end this horrible cycle and was not met with much encouragement or optimism. In a very matter-of-fact way, he said, "This is as good as it gets." I was determined to prove him wrong.

I started researching food as medicine, as an approach to healing my pancreas and digestive system. I incorporated holistic practices like herbal medicine and became more consistent again with my yoga practice. These lifestyle changes helped to manage my stress, which then kept the inflammation down in my body and prevented future pancreas flare-ups. I'm happy to report that I have kept my pancreas in pristine shape, have not been admitted to the hospital again for pancreatitis, and have not had any repeat surgeries in over 15 years. I took agency over my well-being and ended this health crisis that had become such a big part of my life.

In an effort to make yoga a more impactful part of my lifestyle and be able to share this gift with others, I decided to take more intensive training. Through yoga teacher training, I was able to explore the philosophy and history of yoga in order to get a better understanding of why the poses and meditation were having such an impact on my life and well-being.

Once I completed training, I chose to return to the YMCA to teach yoga because I wanted this practice to be accessible to people in my community who were not going to find yoga at a yoga studio. I saw how much it helped me with my physical, mental, and emotional health and was determined to provide others with the exposure to yoga that I was granted through my YMCA membership.

I attribute yoga as the core practice that has helped to build resilience as a nurse and as a Black woman. Incorporating yoga into my lifestyle has given me tools to care for body, mind, and spirit. Yoga has helped me be less reactive and therefore, I believe it matured me emotionally. I was very naive in a lot of things and had some fairly unhealthy patterns in relationships and friendships with over giving and not having healthy boundaries. Learning the foundational yoga philosophies helped me to put things in a different perspective that allowed me to center who I am and how I am in relationship with the world.

From the time we are born, women — especially Black women — are taught to be strong and fiercely independent. There is a strong Black woman's creed that tells us to take care of everyone else first and put everyone's needs ahead of our own. There's almost a pride that comes with being so self-sufficient that you don't need anyone or anything outside of yourself. And for many of us, that belief system carries us through the tough times. While it's important to know your own strength, many Black women like myself reach a breaking point and have to finally learn the art of sacred self-care.

Yoga helped me challenge this belief system of self-sacrifice and started me on a journey of reflection and personal inquiry. Yoga taught me to listen to my body and the signals it sends to slow down and rest. And because I am in a better relationship with my body, I don't have to have a complete system shutdown to signal me to rest. I have learned to be present and mindful of my pancreas by noticing any early signs of digestive distress and responding with the appropriate lifestyle adjustments.

I remember one point in my graduate nursing program, I was still playing superwoman and juggling way too much. I was in school and working full time, had a newborn son that I was nursing, and was not long recovered from my first surgery. So, it should come as no surprise, my pancreas flared up and I was soon facing my second pancreatic cyst and subsequent surgery.

A few years later while in a nursing PhD program, I had started to study and practice yoga more regularly. After recovering from two surgeries, incorporating food as medicine, supplementing with herbal therapy, and regularly practicing yoga and meditation, my overall stressors were the same but my tools for resilience were more intentional and impactful. This shift was proof to me that the yoga practices I was incorporating into my life were essential to keeping me at an optimal level of physical, mental, and spiritual health.

I believed in this holistic approach so much that I began to share these practices in my nursing roles. At the time, I taught at the university and was intentional about teaching simple mindfulness and meditation practices to my students and colleagues. While teaching one particularly challenging graduate course, I had many opportunities to share with my students and colleagues simple mindfulness practices and continued those practices myself.

We talk a lot about burnout in nursing and how to change our work environments so that nurses are less stressed. I sincerely wish that someone had taught me these yoga and mindfulness tools as a nursing student. I'm confident that it would have made a vast difference across the course of my nursing career.

I have had feedback from students who participated in a guided meditation with me come back to me weeks or even years later to share the positive impact it had on them. When someone comments that I have a calming presence, I know in my heart it is because I am practicing yoga in all the ways that matter. Embodying yoga on and off the mat means that you can engage more sincerely with students, patients, and family. Those reflections mean the world to me because I know that many of us healthcare professionals are very pragmatic and scientific see things like yoga as too 'woo-woo'. I'm just grateful to know that a growing number of us are willing to experience it firsthand and decide for themselves how much impact it can have.

Another really significant way that I matured emotionally and spiritually with yoga has been in my role as a parent. I am able to approach parenting situations more strategically because I'm not so reactive. My spiritual practice guides me to take a holistic approach to all aspects of my life, and I try to teach my children this same approach. Now they have a very intentional, thoughtful, and spiritual life. They're not just following along some path because it's the one that was given to them. We have deep conversations about what they believe and why. They take ownership of learning for themselves and take responsibility for their actions. I have had my daughter send me a video showcasing her yoga skills. And I have walked into a room to find my son exploring yoga poses on his own. It warms my heart to see them incorporating this practice in their lives as well.

The most rewarding yoga class of my career thus far has been a class I teach with young Black men. I led a weekly beginner's class to a teenaged basketball team whose coach solicited my assistance hoping yoga would help prevent injuries. We started our journey with exploring the different poses, and they often commented to me or the coach that they could see the changes in their body from week to week.

Once I had their trust a bit more, I decided to incorporate a bit of meditation into our flow. This was important to me because I have a teenage son and know firsthand how crucial the year of isolation in 2020 has impacted their collective mental health. To my surprise, with a generation that values constant stimulation, they embraced the meditation practice immediately. I saw that they were learning as I did on my yoga journey how yoga benefits the body as well as the mind.

I have witnessed the same pattern happening with my extended family members. My mom, aunt, and mother-in-law are all tapped into yoga classes in their communities. They all were introduced to yoga through community centers and YMCA programs geared towards keeping older adults active. Like myself, these strong Black women would not have ventured into a yoga studio to find this practice. Having access to this practice has allowed them to build the resilience needed to be caregivers for their partners and parents without sacrificing their own well-being.

I believe our communities of color truly need yoga classes, yoga-friendly spaces, accessible classes, and teachers who look like them to make yoga feel more acceptable and welcoming. Having the opportunity to experience the peace and calm that comes with a regular yoga practice can help us get past some of our barriers and questions about yoga: Can this be done by Christians? Is this another religion? What is that language they're saying with the poses?

When they discover the phenomenal benefits of yoga to both body and mind, it helps them get past some of those barriers. They discover yoga can be a supplement to your own belief system and practices.

Yoga allows me to become still and centered enough to find a peace that I can't find any other way. In today's fast-paced society that we live in, if you can create sanctuary and find a way to tap into deep peace, you should hold on to that for dear life. My mission to share the benefits of yoga in my community remains strong because I am a testament to how one melanated yogi took agency over her health crisis and came out stronger as a result.

About LaShanda Brown, PhD

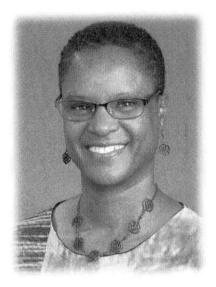

LaShanda Brown, PhD, is a nurse practitioner and yoga teacher who researches nurses' and caregivers' self-care practices with a focus on building and maintaining resilience. Her past research looks historically at the roles of nurses in the community and the impact of their selfless service on the lives they have touched. She is interested in exploring the impact of their service as caregivers on their own personal health and well-being, as well as the benefits of contemplative practices like mindfulness, yoga, meditation, and reflective journaling.

LaShanda teaches yoga and meditation in her community and has witnessed firsthand the positive impact these practices can have on healthcare professionals. She facilitates women's circles and mini-retreats to offer spaces for women to reflect, learn tools for resilience, and form supportive communities.

www.soulcareyoga.net

Chapter 7
Unconditional Yoga:
Loving Our Diversely-Abled Selves

◆━━━━━━◆▸•◀◆━━━━━━▸

Erin Dowd

Perhaps it's true what they say, "the hardest person to love is yourself." Yoga can guide us to love ourselves, yet so many think one has to be in a certain physical condition to do yoga, that yoga isn't for those physically challenged or disabled.

The truth is that no matter one's condition, yoga can be adapted to make it accessible to all people. Sometimes our physical and mental challenges offer opportunities to strengthen our love muscles and soften our hearts.

The Gift of Yoga to Me and My Family

I was born with one foot turned out. Doctors put me in a brace that held my feet in place to turn them forward. They said I should be fine, but on many levels — metaphorically at the very least — I have often felt like I drag one foot behind. I often struggle to keep up with others seemingly more capable, both physically and mentally, in spite of tests indicating me to be near genius in mathematics and spatial and linguistic processing.

Throughout my life, I have gained and lost abilities. Growing up, I had a shelf full of "Most Improved" trophies for participation in neighborhood sports. Although race times improved dramatically, I still usually came in last place and felt the pains of trying so hard. As a teenager, I was diagnosed with early arthritis and told to live a more sedentary life.

I refused. In my early adult years, I continued endeavors into the outdoors for extreme sports. I still love the wild and sensual elements of nature, although putting myself in precarious situations with my challenged body has left me with many injuries.

Yoga was a gift to me. I was introduced to yoga as a child by my librarian grandmother, whose mission in life was to expand libraries' collections to include children's books representing diverse cultures. When I teach children's yoga classes, I share my cherished copy of the first yoga book she purchased, in which pictures of Black and Asian children model the yoga poses.

My grandmother also connected with Lilias Folan's early morning yoga show on PBS. When my cousins, my brothers and I spent time at her house, we would discover her in the living room doing her yoga practice on a towel. She would be rolling around saying how much it helped her feel better every day.

My mother also practiced yoga. When I was a teenager, she introduced me to the value of meditation. Later on, she introduced me to a yoga teacher who offered advanced yoga instruction that was well-balanced with a combination of gentle movement and meditation that was just right for me.

So early on, I learned to breathe and relax through yoga and I loved how it lowered the stress and anxieties so many of us face with the challenges of living in this world.

Initially, I thought that yoga was only for people with an able body and mind. Although somewhat challenged, I was privileged to be able to do the practices offered by my early teachers. I perhaps would have been considered by many to have an advanced yoga practice.

I believe my true advancement began with a backcountry skiing injury. Instead of following the guide's instructions to allow ourselves to just fall over if not flowing easily, I insisted on trying to stay upright and pushed my body in a different direction than my ski was able to go.

I felt a pop in my knee and my face planted in the snow. I lifted my head to breathe and felt my leg dangling in the air behind me. I was unable to stand and had to be lowered in a rescue body wrap and helicoptered off that mountain. The injury left me temporarily disabled with a torn ACL and four other knee-supporting ligaments surgeons recommended repairing.

At that time, I was in an elective college yoga class. I showed up to class with a drop slip, and other students who saw me with my big knee brace and crutches said, "Aww, you're going to have to drop the class!"

But our teacher, Hansa, gave me a big smile and said, "You get to learn modification!" Hansa not only showed me how to practice chair yoga that semester but also became a life-long teacher and guided me in the direction of my career as an Adaptive Yoga Teacher.

One time in Hansa's class while I still had my knee brace, the cool down was a seated forward fold over one leg at a time. I was fine doing this over my functional leg, but when it came time to do the injured leg, as she reminded us to love the leg we were leaning over, my eyes filled with tears. I realized I didn't love all of me.

When faced with imperfection and inability, I didn't love myself. My love of myself was conditional to my ability and my previous patterns of always improving. I began to understand more about unconditional love and started to love myself more wholly.

I was so thankful to be welcomed, even when disabled, to stay and participate in yoga class. At that time, my body hurt more than ever. My stress elevated and being able to practice yoga left me feeling better, both physically and mentally.

I learned to listen not only to the teacher but also to myself. I learned to feel love for myself as I was, no matter my condition. To this day, as my body has gone through numerous other injuries, I keep practicing yoga.

I also now suffer from migraines that mean sometimes enduring so much pain that I have to stay home and reschedule sessions with students. Thankfully, we all adapt as needed.

Doctors have recommended I apply for disability benefits, but with the support of a variety of healing arts, business coaching and family support, I manage an entrepreneurial path working full-time through self-employment that allows me to take breaks to rest when needed.

My ability to go slow has really turned out to be a benefit in terms of working in the world of yoga, because in yoga slow is better. The goal is to slow down, not only the body but especially the mind.

An integrated nervous system, both central and peripheral, and a connection to spirit — these things are accessible to all people. So long as we are alive and breathing, we are able to practice yoga.

It is so fulfilling to adapt yoga for people who are mostly sedentary due to the disabilities they live with and to offer them access to a physical and movement-based yoga practice.

I know a man who is now quadriplegic after a mountain biking accident and was told he would never move again, yet he can now feed himself with his own hands again and has regained movement by doing mind work and retraining his body.

I also work with other high-performing athletes to balance their activity with the stillness and peace of long-held Restorative poses and Yoga Nidra meditations. This calms their active bodies and minds. Many people can go on solo adventures out in the world yet sometimes struggle to come home to self and be able to relax and slow down.

Whether I am doing my own practice or leading another individual or group, I love how yoga brings me to a centered place where I can feel focused and awake to whatever is being experienced, whether desired or not.

I modify the poses for myself and for others as needed. A downward dog pose on the floor can bring pain, but when doing it with hands on a wall, or a table or countertop, a wondrous release can occur in our backs. Standing hero pose can be done seated, or maybe we can be heroes lying on the ground supported with yoga props while doing a Restorative practice.

If I go to most yoga classes being offered in athletic yoga studios in my part of the world — the kind that most mainstream American society think of as yoga — I leave in pain if I don't modify the majority of it. On the flip side, if I do no yoga, I suffer from tightening, weakness, and a hyperactive mind.

They say a long spine is the secret to longevity. Yoga does help lengthen and strengthen the spine. I have to be really careful, though, because I also have spinal stenosis. I am very sensitive to too much movement, so I have to do just the right amount and let it be enough.

Because of the way I practice, doctors, instead of telling me that I should stop doing activity, now say, "Keep doing your yoga. It is helping you."

The most modification I have ever needed was when I was pregnant. My personal yoga practice continued and supported me, but my teaching work needed a long maternity leave both pre- and post-natal.

My body was so challenged that supporting myself and the baby in utero was all I could do. I did the one and only

Restorative pose I could do throughout my entire third trimester. After the baby was born, I leaned on the diaper-changing table for support, until I gradually regained strength doing Moon Salutations.

The baby would watch me and gradually began to mimic me in her own ways. I cherish a video of her and I doing Moon Salutations together with her in a front carrier. I'm going side to side in crescent moon and the other poses in the sequence, as she delightfully moves her head and arms back and forth side to side.

We now have nighttime and morning yoga routines, and with the baby now a toddler, we often vary the routines quite a bit. That's yoga. When we try to repeat an exact prescribed way, it can be overly controlling and not necessarily as yogic anymore. I tell my students, "I know you're doing yoga when you do something different than I say. I know that you're really listening to your body."

My Gift of Yoga to Others

It is common to hear people say, "I can't do yoga, because (fill in the blank/part of me) isn't able." I understand they haven't been offered yet the gift of yoga teachings I received and now give to others. With Adaptive Yoga, everyone is able.

Yoga can serve people with diverse abilities, whether from physical or mental challenges, from injury or illness, and whether temporary or permanent.

Some of the most physically challenged I've known include people living in wheelchairs, some with paralysis, others with missing limbs, and some having impaired senses, such as those with blindness.

I also work with mental challenges, including people of all ages, some with developmental delays, people on the autism spectrum, people with early memory loss and forms of dementia such as Alzheimer's and others.

For all, I offer yoga practices that aim to help us accept and love who we are, how we are, where we are, right here, right now. We go with the flow.

Adaptive Yoga can be adventurous. I don't show up with a prescribed plan for my students other than a plan to adapt as needed for the given students with whom I am working. I include all parts of a very open template of a classic yoga sequence.

We begin with present moment awareness, then set intentions, breathe, warm up, move around all directions possible, bring bilateral awareness to all parts of the body on all sides, and cool down before a final rest and meditation. Easy, and also takes some training to know how to do it with adaptive ways.

After any given practice I lead, it is the smiles and stories shared that make the challenge so worthwhile. Even though I keep trying to give back to them, they also keep giving back to me every time. It's a giving and receiving, a loving exchange and cycle that just keeps going.

One of my students, who was really profound for me to work with, is blind. He had gone to a public yoga class and was told by the teacher to seek out private instruction. I do a lot of private instruction for special groups and also for individuals. He asked for one-on-one work, and we worked together for years.

It was interesting, because it seemed he was so used to touch and being guided hands-on. In the yoga world, we call it an "adjustment" when a teacher touches your body to help you adjust positioning. While adjustments can be safe, I also know many who have actually been hurt by them, so I prefer not to adjust much. I use verbal cues more and try to let students adapt themselves as they feel right.

This student was so courageous to move in space he couldn't see. He listened not only to my direction but also to messages his body gave him to move certain ways, with trust in the playful and creative aspects of the practice.

I loved that he always did his homework. I try to give homework to all my students, although very few report actually doing it. I ask them to practice on their own without me, to learn that yoga is accessible to them at any time whether with or without a teacher present. That's a big lesson to learn that many don't always get to. He was all over it.

He was an excellent student. He came for weekly sessions to learn his new lessons and would practice on his own every day the rest of the week. He advanced so much that he eventually chose to transition into solely wanting guidance with Yoga Nidra meditations, which are also available online for free yet even more powerful when guided by a live teacher in person.

He went from being someone who seemed hesitant with much yoga movement in the beginning to the point that he was confident to move on his own in his own time and then was ready for the meditative practice when he came for his private yoga session.

This was a remarkable accomplishment since meditation is considered to be the ultimate and most powerful part of yoga — to calm the mind and be able to feel the nature of our being.

Not all students are ready for this. I also have experience as a licensed schoolteacher and love adapting yoga for children. They need to move a lot and usually need shorter times for quiet integration.

Regardless of age, there's often a lot of storytelling to carry us through our flow. We adapt not only our movement but also our words in ways that are moving, inspiring, and empowering.

One concern I have is that not only students but also many teachers are perpetuating the myth that yoga is only for able bodies and minds. There is a sense of despair in thinking one is unable to access such a powerful practice that could be made more available to people if more knowledge of how to adapt yoga was included in yoga teacher training programs, as it was in my training with Hansa.

What pains me even more than a student thinking they can't do yoga is when I hear other yoga teachers say they or any one of their students have to take a break from yoga because of an injury. I want to say, "No, don't stop. Show your students that yoga never stops." But they have to learn this for themselves.

My desire is for more teachers to learn to adapt yoga and model this for their students, like the time when I was still teaching mainstream public yoga classes at a studio and showed up to teach with my broken wrist in a cast. The students got to see how the yoga could still be done, just different, but still "Oh, so good!"

The Gift of Love for All

We are wise to learn to receive support. We don't have to go it alone. We are in this together. While we may want to work towards increasing independence and self-sufficiency, we are even better when we join together to nurture connections in community. This helps it feel easier to relax and love what is.

The gifts of yoga and also experiences with other healing arts help us to love our body, mind and spirit, and to increase not only our own but also societal resilience, strength, and flexibility.

Love breathing easier. All living bodies can do the most important part—breathing. If we're living, we're breathing. The number one thing about yoga is to work with our breath and present moment awareness.

Love being bold, bright, beautiful, strong, smart, and sensual, regardless of pose-ability. When we do it together, it can feel like a heightened power of our multiplied and shared energy. Then to also be able to do it alone in our own way can be even another kind of energy to feel one's own power and know it is enough.

I have one student who has never moved anything below his head on his own, yet he is always smiling and makes eye contact the minute you see him. He sends positive vibrations to the group by simply being there and expressing his happiness.

In the meditations and in the way we do or don't move, we can reflect on the elements of nature, including other animals and parts of our natural environment. This helps us to come back and reflect on our human nature and what it is to live a life in which we all struggle yet also triumph.

We all have been wounded or struggled in some way. We survive it, get through it, and we grow. Then we can go even further — beyond surviving and thriving to do even more, to contribute and give back to community.

Those who were born with, or at some point acquired, disabilities very much long to be included more, as they are so often otherwise left out, and community yoga helps to lower the feelings of stress and isolation.

It can be challenging to feel loved by others and to feel love for self when labeled and feeling different. Yoga can help.

Having a yoga teacher inform me that I could still practice yoga, even disabled, was the greatest gift. I learned that the teachings of yoga are unconditional, universal, and can be practiced by literally anyone.

We modify the practice, not the person. I've heard it said, "We teach people, not poses." Poses can be modified to any degree or can be solely visualized. Poses can also be left out altogether. For instance, you don't have to do the shoulder stand, commonly known as the "queen of all poses" and considered by many yoga teachings to be essential. This kind of inversion is better avoided by those with spinal conditions and certain other health concerns.

It's also not necessary to lie down for a closing meditation. To say "no" is part of loving. Comfort and safety are important.

I heard once that when you roll up your yoga mat, that is when your yoga practice really begins. Yoga practice is meant to be applied to life.

Actually, I rarely use a mat. It's just one of many optional props, not required. All you need is a breathing body and a space where you can be comfortable.

Partial disability, pregnancy and parenting are perhaps the most challenging experiences I've had yet. Birthing and bonding with a child has been the greatest blessing I've known, although it often can be stressful.

Stress for any reason makes life harder to manage, and the right adapted yoga practice helps to lower the stress and bring back more laughter and joy. We must be friendly with *all* our feelings, desired or not.

When feelings are hard to recognize, we can notice the positioning of our hands and feet, the expressions on our faces, the thoughts in our heads, and under relaxed shoulders feel the movement of our hearts. May we follow where our hearts lead us.

To desire a "regular" or "normal" life or to think there is a "normal yoga" may be a natural inclination, yet with a dive deeper into what exactly is normal, we usually discover there is no such thing.

Appreciating my grandmother's inspiration as an early promoter of the Civil Rights Movement to include people of all races and ethnicities, I hope to also see more diversity in yoga by including people with diverse abilities benefiting from Adaptive Yoga, loving themselves and feeling able to contribute to the world we live in and create.

I believe that ultimately we are all more similar than we are different, and yoga is really about the unity that embraces our diversity. As they say, "We are all one." All loved.

About Erin Dowd, E-RYT

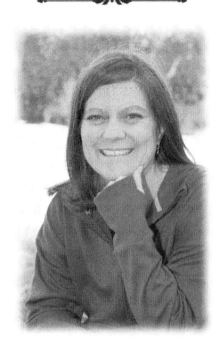

(Credit for Erin Dowd's photos: JC Ash Photography.)

Erin Dowd, E-RYT, was introduced to yoga as a child. Her love for yoga grew even more when she discovered how yoga serves those disabled. She learned chair yoga after her own injury and then continued to learn how to adapt the practice for literally anyone.

She began teaching yoga in 2007 and is an E-RYT now serving individuals and groups in private sessions. Her favorite part of teaching is seeing the smiles on people's faces when they practice.

You can reach Erin at

Facebook erin.dowd.31 or turtlesther@gmail.com

Chapter 8
The Power of Rest:
Healing Magic for Midlife & Menopause

◆▶·◀◆

Cindi Buenzli Gertz

Rest saved my life.

You might think that as a yoga teacher, I'd say, "*yoga* saved me." But no, I credit rest — one of the most underrated and underwhelming gifts we can give ourselves — with liberating my life, especially during peri-menopause.

Resting and releasing are a vital part of yoga, but ironically, I struggled the most with learning how to truly and deeply let go. I understood the concept of *doing* yoga, but the resting aspect of it took much longer for me to grasp. When I finally discovered it, yoga set me on a proper course to healing, but I still shudder to think about how difficult my life would be now if I hadn't found yoga or rather if yoga hadn't found me.

I'm telling this story during a time of massive upheaval around the globe while simultaneously navigating the messy in-between we call midlife.

In 2020, I turned 50 and became a crone, not a dirty word to my ear, but one of reverence symbolizing the wisdom years, as I crossed the threshold into menopause. Our son, Ray, graduated from high school, and we packed him off to college to start a new adventure of his own. We taught our youngest, our daughter Helen, how to drive, a transition that nudged us closer to *the* empty nest.

But I would not go quietly into the next chapter of my life.

I celebrated these landmark occasions not with a sense of dread around aging, shriveling up, or becoming invisible, like so many midlife women fear, but rather enthusiasm. I felt healthier and more vibrant than ever — full of joy, wonder, gratitude, abundance, and excitement for the future. As I danced through the mystery of menopause, I felt ready to expand, grow, and imagine infinite possibilities for the second half of my life — a life where I could live to be 100 or more!

This kind of vibrancy eluded me in my younger years. Before yoga entered my life — over 20 years ago — I veered toward burnout with breakneck speed. I came from a family rooted in a very strong work ethic. I paid for college on my own, and while I took a full course load, I often held multiple jobs at a time to make ends meet.

When I graduated cum laude, I headed into the nonprofit world to be a helper and make a difference. I kept right on working. And working. And working some more. Pushing, pleasing, and perfecting through the first seven years of my professional life, I skimped on my self-care in every possible way. I saw zero value in taking breaks and getting enough rest.

Long hours, poor food choices, no rest or relaxation, my mind always moved and so did my body — like a machine. Except I forgot to maintain the sacred instrument housing my soul. I forgot to hit the off switch and power down on a regular basis.

I busied myself taking care of everyone else, but not me. Employed first by the National MS Society (Michigan) and then by Big Brothers Big Sisters of the Western Upper Peninsula, I kept saying "yes" to work. I kept saying "yes" to producing, pleasing, and perfecting.

At the age of 28, I developed Seasonal Affective Disorder. I started to fumble, barely able to get myself out of bed and to work before 10 o'clock in the morning most days. I endured horrific headaches after carrying my work stress to bed with me and grinding my teeth in the night.

As a child, I had responded naturally to chronic seasonal allergies by resting. But as an adult, I *forgot* how to rest and take care of myself. My allergies worsened and left my immune system on overdrive, completely overwhelmed and weakened. As a result, I experienced one cold after another.

The colds always started in late summer and raged on for months until I developed a full-blown sinus infection by the holidays. This cycle went on year after year. Still, I kept pushing.

I kept pushing until one time after a work trip I thought I just had to take. This time, my body said — no screamed — "ENOUGH!"

During the winter of 1999, I found myself grounded at the Detroit International Airport after a storm dumped over 12 inches of snow across the state. Desperate to get home, I thought it brilliant to rent a car with two college students and drive back to the Upper Peninsula, a 10-hour journey in good weather. Of course, sick with a cold again, I was in no shape to drive. Truth be told, I don't remember most of the ride as I slept in the back seat while two young men, complete strangers to me, took the wheel.

Looking back at my foolishness, I know I'm lucky to be alive. My wakeup call came the day after I survived that unbelievable trip home. As I stood in our local grocery store looking at the cans of processed soup and trying to decide which one would nourish me best (insert a snicker here and maybe an eye roll, too), the world closed in on me. The edges of my vision started turning black, a circle of light grew smaller and smaller and smaller...

...and the next thing I knew, I was on the floor, waking up, right in the middle of the canned goods aisle.

Fortunately, my brother, Steve, had been standing right next to me. A big strong guy with the tenderest of hearts, he picked me up, carried me to the bench at the front of the store, and called my husband, Michael, on the intercom. Shortly after I had passed out, they took me to the doctor who put me on a week's bed rest. Although I wouldn't understand it for years to come, this event marked a huge turning point for me.

Around the time of my wake-up call, a volunteer, who I worked with, with a very keen eye that I can see in hindsight, suggested that I try yoga. "Pah," I thought. I thanked her kindly and put the brochure in my drawer where it sat for months. However, the thought kept niggling at me, and eventually I started my first yoga class.

What struck me most — I still remember — was the relief I felt when my first teacher, Connie Hawley, told me I could rest, that I could let go. When I tell this part of the story out loud, it never fails to bring tears to my eyes — I think because it pains me to remember how cruelly I treated myself, how easily I said "no" to me back then.

That day after class, I skipped the two blocks back to my office, which was near the yoga studio. My naïve mind rejoiced that I would be able to focus better and do more in less time because of doing yoga. I laugh now because those of us who "do" yoga know that's true on one level. Yoga does help us focus and feel clearer, which then affects the efficiency of everything we do.

Yet, my intention completely missed the mark.

Yoga still wasn't about me and my health; it wasn't about taking care of the sacred vessel of my body. It was about everything outside of me. It was still about doing. It was still about working... pushing, pleasing, perfecting.

I had a long way to go before I understood *being*.

That day, I received permission from my teacher to rest, but years passed before I would grant myself that same grace. Admittedly, relaxing and resting were the hardest parts of yoga practice for me to learn and to really get. In fact, I almost gave up on yoga during the first year of my practice.

Busy again, my husband and I were only married a year and wrapped up in the details of starting a life together. We had just moved to a new town, just rented our first house together, and both just started new jobs. I came home one day completely overwhelmed and declared to Michael, "I'm too busy. I don't have time for yoga right now." To which he said, "Don't you know that's when you need it the most?"

This moment marked another huge turning point for me. What he said sunk in. I recommitted to finding a new teacher in my new town, and the very next week, *she* walked into *my* place of work. In the building to check out available spaces, she introduced herself to me and said she was looking for a new yoga studio location. I don't think the universe could have spoken any louder. And once again, yoga found me.

I studied with Sue Stephens for a year when she invited me to consider teacher training so that I could help her out with the community's growing interest in yoga. I attended Kripalu Center for Yoga and Health in the Berkshires of Massachusetts and earned my teacher certificate. At that point, I had no idea the changes that would take place in my life, let alone the transformations of the many lives of my students to follow.

Within a few years, we moved to Wisconsin, bought our first home, and grew our family to four, plus so many pets, we felt outnumbered. Life got much fuller. I managed our home and cared for our children's daily needs while Michael taught full-time at the high school. I juggled homeschooling with serving my community in various volunteer roles and opened my first yoga studio.

Yep, I was crazy-busy again. Once more, my body howled. This time, I landed in the ER doubled over with pain in my abdomen. A large cyst, which stymied the doctors, had formed in my pelvic cavity. Surgery was suggested, but this time, I listened to my body. I turned to my yoga tools.

I had recently been introduced to restorative yoga by a fellow teacher. I fell in LOVE. The yoga props gently held and supported me in various restorative poses that I had learned. I took a holistic approach, combining restorative and intuitive practices that opened my body, heart, and mind and allowed me to heal without surgery.

Soon after, I heard that Judith Hanson Lasater, a renowned yoga mentor, would be leading a restorative teacher training in Minneapolis, just an hour from my home. I jumped at the chance and earned my Relax & Renew Teacher Certificate. I have continued to train with Judith both in person and online ever since.

Once certified, I specialized in teaching restorative yoga to other women who had also burned out and broken down. While guiding these women, I deepened my own practice of rest and relaxation. My awakening slowly continued to unfold over many years.

And the shifts have been enormous.

I measure the health of my moods and the intensity of my Seasonal Affective Disorder (SAD) by how many days I just want to crawl back into bed and bury my head in the covers.

In years past, I felt drawn toward this abyss most days. This year, I counted only two days where depression threatened to drag me under. And I won't credit SAD for those days. A family member fell seriously ill, and I was naturally and authentically grieving, not reacting chemically to a lack of light and vitamin D.

I still get the occasional headache, but now I have the tools of rest and relaxation to help me get through it. I no longer get colds like I did in the past, where they lasted for weeks on end. I contract one or two colds a year, and they last anywhere from one to three days, possibly a week at most. And the best news: I haven't had a sinus infection in 18 years!

Now when late summer comes around, I barely notice my allergies. Are they gone? No, I don't think so. I used to sequester myself to the basement to escape the allergens, but by doing so, I also separated myself from my family.

These days, I'm not pushing through. I'm saying "yes" to my self-care and no longer need to retreat to the dampness and dark. Even though the ragweed season is lasting three weeks longer on average, I'm able to breathe freely and easily, and I have energy for my everyday activities.

Probably the most profound impact of rest came during my peri-menopause journey, which lasted 10 years. Maybe I should say the permission to rest had finally impacted my life at the deepest level.

I went through the ups and downs of peri-menopause like most women, and there came a time when my hot flashes surged. Night sweats drenched me. I felt so foggy-brained from disrupted sleep that I could barely think straight. I felt exhausted.

I chose to rest. And rest deeply.

I practiced restorative yoga every day. And finally with a little encouragement from friends, I gave myself a six-month sabbatical. By this time, I had been a self-employed yoga teacher with my own studio for many years, so the only one to sign off on this break, this rest, was me. I had to grant myself permission.

I acknowledge that not every woman has the means to do this, and I feel grateful beyond measure that I do. I'm dedicated to teaching women how to take their own mini-sabbaticals during their days, if weeks or months are not an option. I will teach restorative yoga to every woman who will give herself that same permission. If she can't give herself permission yet, I consider it my job to hold that belief for her until she can.

During my sabbatical, I supported myself and a very small circle of women that I had been working with privately. I didn't plan, promote, or promise any new classes. I became very still; I'd had lots of practice by then. I immersed myself more deeply into restorative yoga. I put the call out to the divine feminine to guide me. I invited in her presence. Then, I waited and listened. I awakened to her song and the scene she painted for me.

I saw vividly, a circle of women swirling around in my mind. I recalled a dream I'd had years before that suddenly made complete sense. Early in my marriage, I had dreamt of a symbol that appeared to be a flower. Glowing in hues of burnt orange, tangerine and coral, the petals folded around each other reminding me of the shape of the vulva, the vagina, the yoni. At that time, when I awoke from dream, I drew a picture of it that I still have; the dream felt that powerful.

During my sabbatical, I also heard "start a circle of women who can go through peri-menopause and menopause together." With every fiber of my being, I felt the idea of a sisterhood of celebration, a new legacy rising up — one that could break the silence around the most potent but undervalued and overlooked time of a woman's life. I wanted to lean into, not push away, this rite of passage.

Now, I'm a midlife midwife for women. I bring the divine feminine into their yoga and self-care practices, their relationships, their work, and their lives. I help them navigate the unknowns of peri-menopause, menopause, and midlife with more ease, calm, grace, and confidence. I help them birth themselves into the next iteration of who they're becoming.

And it's *magical*.

Countless times, I've said to students past and present, "There's no magic pill or bullet. The magic is IN the practice."

Why did it take me so long to find that magic? Why did I forget how to rest like I easily had as a child? I believe my perception of time got in the way. The mantra, "I don't have enough time" ran through my head constantly. I lived in scarcity mode for years and heard what I call the "4 Not Enoughs" repeatedly from myself, my middle-aged friends, and my female students . . .

not enough time,
not enough energy,
not enough money,
and every variation of what boils down to . . .
I'm not enough.

Here's the secret I didn't know back then: Every time I practiced restorative yoga, I shattered another limiting belief around the scarcity mentality. I replaced the mindset of lack with one of abundance. Here's why I think that is.

Restorative yoga teaches us to support the body — to open, to release, and to receive. We *receive* restorative yoga; we don't *do* restorative yoga. We receive, fill up, and experience a sense of abundance every time we practice this form of yoga. However, by the time we women reach midlife, we've become expert do-ers, and we're depleted. I've helped not only myself but also many other midlife women undo the *doing* and relearn *receiving* through resting and restorative yoga.

Several years ago, I made a discovery that helped me understand why rest is so very important for the midlife woman. First, I observed this habit in myself. Then I started seeing it in women all around me. Most women I know, women like yourself, engage in two key behaviors that keep them from putting their own self-care above anything else.

First, I see women holding the bigger picture for their families and communities and taking this view into account with almost every decision they make. Second, I see women anticipating the needs of everyone else around them, unfortunately, at the cost of foreseeing their own desires. When I share this in the talks that I give, I always see heads nodding in recognition.

And holy hell, when I hear myself say it out loud, I realize that every woman likely requires a whole lot more rest than she's getting. More rest than she thinks she needs. And worse yet, more than she thinks she deserves.

A great paradox confounds me. The stage of life when a woman needs the most rest coincides *exactly* with the time she is least able to make space for it. I see women in midlife sandwiched between raising children, reaching the height of a career, managing a home, volunteering in their communities, and caring for aging parents. No wonder so many women feel there isn't any time to spare for themselves. Then, peri-menopause arrives on the scene at this same crossroads.

The passion that burns in me now, like the hot flash rising up from my feet to my crown or moving from the inner depths of my being outward, calls me to help other women say "yes" to themselves and feel alive again. I aim to help women thrive throughout midlife and menopause. I strive to help them create the body and being they desire to carry them through the rest of their lives.

Resting taught me to *not* push away, push down, or push through. That transformation helped me move through midlife and into menopause with more grace and ease. As I sank deliciously into my restorative yoga props during my sabbatical, resting showed me how to lean into the "pause" in peri-menopause.

I invite you to do the same. Savor this time. Bathe in it; soak in it. Let the creative juices of your waning menstrual flow move in new directions allowing you to manifest the body, being, and life you desire most. Let yourself wonder and dream. Remember my dream of the flower? I kept the drawing of that mystical symbol, considering what the heck it meant and always believing that I'd find out some day. I finally realized the image represented my own and every woman's awakening and unfolding. The divine feminine awoke my receptivity, intuition, and trust. I remembered to listen to my own inner wisdom.

I hope to help you and every other midlife woman see that you hold the power, that you alone hold the key to saying "yes" to yourself. I provide the space and show you how to turn the key to unlock your infinite possibility. Like my teacher did for me so many years ago, I can give you permission to rest; you'll have to do your part to accept or receive that invitation. Nothing will miraculously change to create the space you need for your self-care practices. You need to give yourself permission, and then you'll see:

The magic's in the practice.

Vibrantly Yours,
Cindi Buenzli Gertz

About Cindi Buenzli Gertz

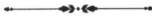

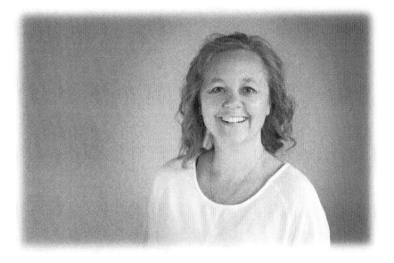

Cindi Buenzli Gertz helps women awaken the divine feminine within themselves so they can move through midlife and transition to menopause with more peace, clarity, grace, and vibrancy. A Certified Kripalu Yoga Teacher and Relax & Renew Trainer, she shows women how to rest deeply and breakthrough the habits of pushing, pleasing, and perfecting — a struggle she overcame in her own life.

In her women's circles, classes, and events, she also draws on her passions for the Earth, holistic living, dream insight, and the arts — powerful aides in her own healing journey — to design transformational experiences. As creator of the Vibrant Woman Program, Cindi inspires her midlife sisters to design their own joyful journey, come alive again, and thrive with abundance.

I'd love to stay in touch and hear your questions, thoughts, and dreams. Sign up for my free Joyful Journey, a short weekly love note that's intended to uplift, teach, and inspire a shift, at this link: http://bit.ly/joyful-journey.

DEATH WISDOM

Chapter 9
Beauty for Ashes
Surviving Trauma When Faith and Joy Became Real

⬥⬥•⬥⬥

Angie Merritt

Trauma

A young man shot another young man. He died, bleeding out after gurgling in surprise, "Hey, you shot me bro!" Have you ever really thought about what it would be like to be the mother of that young man, who bled out on the floor next to the broken Christmas cactus that he knocked over in falling? Or have you ever thought what it might be like to be the mother of the killer, protecting his girlfriend behind him from the fury of an aggressor on drugs, who stood between them and the door to outside? Have you ever thought of what it might be like to be the mother of both, and love them both?

I am that mother and this is my story of how I survived this traumatic event, and how I went on the thrive in my 60s and 70s. So how do I, twenty plus years later, in my seventies, lead my life in peaceful, joyful enthusiasm, serving others as a yoga teacher and helping my small Southern community learn better eating habits? People are shocked when they learn my back story. I will attempt to share some of the pieces that got me here. My deep Christian faith and beliefs got me through those awful days and my experience with yoga, Ayurveda, and meditation helped restore my joy.

By joy, I mean a happy vibration down to my very cells. It is my hope that the yogis reading this will gain some understanding of how Christianity can be a deep helpful faith and that Christians might come to understand the power of yoga to deepen their ability to be Christlike.

I was not at home when my younger son shot his older brother. I arrived home after the police had been called and after the ambulance had carried away the body. The neighbors stood around watching from their yards as all this unfolded.

That New Year's Day in 1998, I sat outside alone on the steps to the carport, but no one came to comfort me. The police were in the house doing their crime scene investigation. I was in shocked disbelief. I had two thoughts.

One thought was that I had to be a terrible mother to allow this to happen. The second thought I had sitting alone in the cold was that God had to have a big lesson for the good of many from this because this was beyond as bad as I could imagine.

First a little more of my backstory.

The whole fall had been miserable and continually becoming worse. I was recovering from failed marriage number two and a related major financial setback. I was in high menopause with greatly disturbed sleep, hot flashes, muddled thoughts, and depression. I struggled all fall, going through the motions of normal activities with great effort and lack of interest in anything. Even my choral group preparing for our Christmas concert brought no pleasure.

And I had a new principal at the high school where I juggled three job titles. I really was not up to everything I needed to do. I could barely come up from the deep well of depression to say hello to friends. The principal noticed and we had problems.

My 21-year-old had been a prickly person since his early teens. He was depressive, had learning disabilities and worst of all, he had bullied his younger brother into being his servant for years. I had found no way to turn this around. He had turned 21 and was old enough to buy alcohol and it unbalanced his chemistry and made him a bit aggressive.

He was bi-polar, but this was a later discovery as husband number one hadn't shared his own diagnosis.

My 17-year-old had problems of his own. He also had learning disabilities, asthma and acted out at school, mostly in reaction to the abuse by his brother. He had been expelled. He was trying to get his life together. He was working with Vocational Rehabilitation Counseling and had a job, a girlfriend, finished his GED, and was taking welding at the Community College.

Our three stories converged here, leaving one dead, one in jail for murder, and one with a shattered heart, wondering how I could go on.

Faith
Clinging to the Story

I expected deep lessons to come from this tragedy as promised in God's word. The deep lesson I learned is that God is good all the time and if I don't think so at any given moment, I just haven't got the whole picture. If the term "God" makes you uncomfortable, substitute Higher Power, Goddess, the Divine, or Universal Consciousness or whatever makes you comfortable. I will continue to use God because it is so easy to spell. I do deeply want you to know that God is on your side, loving you all the time, but it takes some cooperation on our part to reap blessings.

It may not look like a big deal to you, but the timing of this incident and how God prepared me, was to me, evidence that I was loved. It moved me from intellectually consenting to the goodness of God to a state of being totally convinced.

An old friend called me to get my address to send a Christmas card and hearing in my voice that I was in bad shape, invited me to a mountain vacation after Christmas. We had a wonderful time, walking through the snow, swimming in the indoor pool, cooking homemade soup, and dipping in the jacuzzi. This was the between Christmas and that New Year's Day of my son's death.

During that week, I had time to do a personal Bible study on Spiritual Warfare, for when the world seems to be stacked against you. When I arrived home to a death and a jailing of my two precious sons, I knew how I should respond, not that it didn't take everything I had to get up and make it through every day. I felt like I had direct instructions from God. "Therefore, take up the whole armor of God, that you may be able to withstand in the evil day, and having done all, to stand." Ephesians 6:13 New Kind James Version (NKJV) The goal is to use our spiritual resources to create our story of having all the pieces of armor we need from our Christian understanding to be able to stand in even the worst circumstances. First, keep putting on our story, and then we become active in concern for others. Just stand. Be concerned for others. Don't be totally focused on yourself and what happened to you.

I leaned into God through my grief. My days were hard to get through, but I continued day by day. I read psalms; things weren't going so well for David, who wrote many of the psalms. Mad King Saul was chasing him around the wilderness trying to kill David, God's anointed next king, and David could praise the Lord so well we still read his words. I sang on the praise and worship team that very first Sunday and every Sunday after that. When I sing God's praise, I do it with my whole being, body, mind, and spirit. Christians say that God inhabits the praises of his people. It allows God's presence to be more fully felt. My experience during worship is that I can ask my questions and receive answers.

I read Job. Job lost everything, all his children and his health. Job was told by his wife to curse God and die, but he would not. He had three friends who, while they were not much of a comfort, they stayed there with him. He finally found peace when he began to pray for others. Every week I attended two house churches, which are smaller study groups, and a Bible study. So, I put myself where people could stand by me. Figuratively, I stood and I prayed for others. In accordance with my hunger, I even ate as an act of surrender and obedience, rather than by the clock, as suggested in the Bible study on weight loss I was attending.

The most valuable thing I learned about grief is that each precious memory has to be dealt with separately. We have to say goodbye to the twenty-one-year-old, as well as the cute little four-year-old, sitting on the pumpkin in his red shirt and overalls. Each has an emotional, yet physical bond in our electromagnetic body that must be broken, releasing a chemical wash that floods our brain, which we experience as a deep wave of grief. This is short lived, lasting only seconds. If we just ride the wave, we do better than if we resist.

The grief process takes as long as it takes, but we are not sentenced to stay there forever. Death is part of life. If we expect something different, we just add to our suffering.

Losing your "loser" story can free you to be who you were created to be and ready you to serve in ways that you are especially equipped to serve. What is a "loser" story? We each create our own story that narrates how our life unfolds.

If you frame your story with you as a loser, a victim, then you will live your life as a loser, a victim. If you frame your story to see yourself as a winner, then you are the winner.

I had to forgive myself for being the mother who allowed this to happen to her two children. I had to develop the compassion for myself to allow myself to understand that as a mother in difficult circumstances, I had done the best I could. I learned to live in compassion, understanding that we are all doing the best we can. Eventually we may reach the point where we are just present, aware of the moment without our story, but in the meantime, we need to choose our story from what allows for our growth.

I came to understand that this was not just my story. I was a support character in my oldest son's story. It was his life, his death. And that maybe it was God's mercy to take him earlier than we would expect. He was going to have a life with a lot of unhappiness, maybe even misery. He had accepted Jesus and been baptized, due to a girlfriend getting him into church and early training, and that is supposed to be comforting. While most Christians believe heaven is the next step, being totally convinced that God is good, I can leave those decisions to God.

I learned that thoughts are my responsibility and how to work with them. A verse that I consider my life verse is Romans 12:2 (NKJV) "Do not be conformed to this world, but be transformed by the renewing of your mind, that you may prove what *is* that good and acceptable and perfect will of God." It tells me three things. One, I don't have to think what my culture thinks. Two, I can renew my mind. I learned to look at my thoughts and adjust my attitude, taking my part of the responsibility. We all experience the same emotions, but we can determine how we interact with them.

And third is what God has in mind for me is good. It is acceptable and it is perfect. What we go through, our individual life experiences can shape us to be ready to receive and deliver God's plan for our lives. I certainly wouldn't have picked to go through that time in my life, or my two first marriages, but I learned to renew my mind, look at myself with thoughts of the changes I could make, and to be resilient and contented in the moment.

Joy
Surrendering into Grace

Ten years later, I began to attend yoga classes at the local gym. The teachers weren't trained. One had memorized a yoga DVD. One watched YouTube. But yoga itself is powerful. Yoga began to bring me the gift of greater mindfulness and connection to body. Soon after I began my yoga practice, I realized that if I overeat, I will be uncomfortable. Not earth shattering, I know, but I had begun to live more fully in my body.

Later I noticed that when I got called down for something at work, I experienced a dropping into my gut and a realization that I needed to ride it out so I wouldn't react with anger. I could listen to what they had to say instead of jumping in with what I thought was right. I was an English as a Second Language teacher in a school system with few English learners. Administrators' views, educationally and culturally, were often at odds with my view of the needs of my students. This dropping into my gut puzzled me for quite a while until I learned more about the chakras. Our first chakra is where we experience vulnerability. If we become aware of our fear at that level, the energy is acknowledged and doesn't run up our chakras to be expressed as shame, or anger, or lies.

I am in the process of opening my throat chakra. I love to sing but my voice had dropped to a second alto or tenor range and I had prayed to get my voice back. I was also very reluctant to say what I thought in many situations, although I have plenty of thoughts. It may be from having been raped as a young teen and not feeling free to tell, or even knowing that I should tell. It may be from being a woman before women were welcome to talk, especially in church. Many times I would say what was on my mind only to be ignored in favor of what the next man said, even if it was less pithy. It may be that I was just out of step with my culture. I know that it is also connected to telling my grief.

I added fish pose to the yoga classes I taught because one of my students had thyroid issues and I thought it would help. I felt the heat of opening at the base of my neck for months. My voice restored to its clear lovely alto range and I began the journey toward telling my truth. Writing this story is part of that.

I became a yoga teacher. I began reluctantly, just Level 1, sixteen hours on the way to the required 200 hours. I was called in by my pastors and told it was not a good idea. They did get me a DVD of Christian yoga, but I wasn't impressed with Hebrew music and new names for poses. They wouldn't allow me to teach yoga at the church for fear I would convert people to Hinduism. I could not do that even if I tried. Hinduism is interesting, but since I did not have a spiritual void, I didn't need it. But I was afraid that yoga would take me away from my spiritual foundation, so I approached it very cautiously. I didn't know it would open a much deeper understanding.

One idea I learned to respect is that our western minds tend to think in "either-or" terms, while eastern minds tend to think in "yes, and" terms. I teach yoga and often share its concepts with Bible verses to meet my students where they are.

As I learned more, I was very much drawn to yoga's power to physically and emotionally heal and that it is a spiritual practice helpful to anyone of any faith. As a child, I had wanted to become a medical missionary. I never wanted to become a medical practitioner of any description, but here was my path to become what I had always desired, a healer, working with body, mind, and spirit as well as energy and wisdom.

I added meditation when I found enough resources to learn. I am from a small town in Eastern North Carolina where I am basically the only yoga teacher for miles around.

Meditation has been great for training my brain to be more focused. With meditation, our default mind, the one that jumps around worrying about the past and future, learns to become quiet and more obedient. A focused mind is a happy mind. Meditation allows space for intuition to come forth. In my seventies, I am focused, creative, and not nearly as forgetful as my peers. I am the happiest, most fulfilled and purpose driven I have been in my life.

Yoga grows the spirit within as we are able to lose ego by staying in the present moment, from catching and examining our thoughts and staying connected with our heart and gut brains. As I got more unified in body, mind, and spirit, I became more aware of the energy, the 'prana' in yoga, the 'chi' in Qigong and Tai Chi, the Holy Spirit in Christianity. With time, intention, and practice, our frequency, our personal vibration changes to be aligned with God's loving kindness talked about in the Old Testament, and we live within that vibration, in a state of grace. Living in that grace, allowed me to become more fully feminine, embracing the more receptive, creative side of God. I appreciate the Divine Feminine as the creative energy within us and all things.

Along the yogic path, I discovered self-care and Ayurveda, the sister science of yoga that brings health to us by helping us stay in balance within our own personal makeup and within the daily and seasonal cycles of the earth. So now I eat weeds and walk barefoot on the ground. Ayurveda helps us to be more receptive to the intelligence of our bodies, in constant observation of our condition, and to adjust our self-care as needed. Mostly, I eat whole fresh foods as organic as I can manage and do a few herbs, sometimes. I do daily self-care practices, such as tongue scraping, oil self-massage, walking in nature, and meditation. I am extremely healthy and not on any medications.

Just so you don't leave wondering, my younger son had a court hearing where it was decided he had acted in self-defense. He eventually finished his welding and plumbing certificates. He married the girlfriend. They have two children. He works as a farm equipment mechanic. He has had an emotionally hard time, which I wish weren't so, but he functions and works hard.

My shattered heart is still here within me, and I can fall into deep grief quickly for those few seconds, especially when I tell this tale, which I seldom do. It is a specific tender spot somewhere in my heart chakra throat area. Opening the throat chakra to tell my story is part of the healing. Perhaps it is my gift to give. My vulnerability opens others to their vulnerability and can be very healing. I told my story to a Christian ladies' retreat in Nicaragua and sixty ladies rose to their feet crying and hugging everyone in the room. It was a sweet time.

Mostly I am resilient, resourceful, easygoing, curious, creative, and open. I am in an up spiral of growth — even at my age — becoming that crone, that elder, that guru. Even if my circle is small, it is increasingly sweet. I wanted to write my story to crystalize what my message is from it. I hope my story has some value for you.

In India, they describe different styles of faith by comparing how a baby monkey holds onto its mother for dear life as she leaps to where she is going, but a baby kitten surrenders trustingly as mama cat takes her by the nape to move her.

Both methods demonstrate faith appropriate to the situation. I have moved from baby monkey faith of Christianity in a desperate time in my life to kitten faith, surrendering to loving wisdom as I have grown and become more whole through yoga.

About Angie Merritt

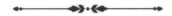

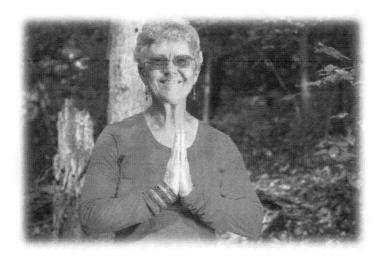

Although Angie Merritt lives in the house in which she was raised, in a poverty pocket of the Bible belt, she has always been fascinated by the cultures, foods, and beliefs of other places and epochs. She has proved her resilience throughout life but has really transformed her health and the boundaries of her life since retiring from teaching.

Now in her 70s, she is the cofounder of Food Cures U, teaching wellness from the kitchen to her community as well as online. She is also the founder of Joyful Vitality Yoga and Health Practices, teaching Chi-infused yoga and leading her life-changing program, Joyful Vitality Lifestyle Journey, a dynamic group experience for empowering health improvement through embodied self-care.

Contact her at JoyfulVitalityYoga@gmail.com or Joyful Yoga with Angie | Facebook for Yoga videos and to sign up for a free 40-minute Thrive Train Strategy Session.

Chapter 10
Grief, Growth, and Sobriety

Michelle Ann Collins

"You've always had the power… "
— Glinda, the Good Witch, *Wizard of Oz*

Watching the *Wizard of Oz* with my mom was a childhood joy. I loved singing with the munchkins and skipping back and forth in front of the TV, pretending I was following the yellow brick road.

"I want to go to Oz!" I cried to my mom.

"You don't need to venture so far from home, Missy. Everything you need is right here," she said, hugging me to her and gently setting me on her lap. I wanted to be Dorothy, singing and dancing down the yellow brick road with her friends. I begged my mom for a flying monkey, and when she had to refuse, I was in tears. Attempting to comfort me, she tried to explain the important lessons from Dorothy's journey, but nothing helped. Especially the part where Dorothy learns that the power to fulfill her heart's desire was with her all along. I wasn't ready for such a lesson at that time.

As a small consolation prize for the lack of a flying monkey, I did receive a pair of ruby slippers. When I wore my small sparkly red shoes, I tapped my heels together trying to make magic. When I failed to fly on a broomstick or create a bubble I could soar around in, I cried in frustration, "Mom, I can't do anything!" Gently placing her beautifully manicured hand in the middle of my chest, my mom said, "Sweetie, you can do anything you want to do, you have everything you need inside of you." At the time, I pictured a flying monkey inside my chest; I was very confused.

"Mom, that doesn't make any sense!" I said, frustrated.

"Remember what Glinda said?" my mom asked.

"She had to learn it for herself. If Glinda had told her that, Dorothy wouldn't have believed her."

"So right now, Honey," my mom cooed, trying to soothe me, "you may not understand, but someday you will." My mom knew that finding gratitude was the key to having everything my heart desired. She knew and wanted me to learn that, like Dorothy, everything I ever needed was already inside me.

My mom was the thread that weaved the entire fabric of my life together. She was the embodiment of kitchen table wisdom. Growing up, and even when I was supposed to be a grown-up with my own kids, I sat at her table late into the evening pouring out my heart, sharing my deepest fears and desires. Her wisdom and loving presence were all I needed to handle anything. Conversations with my mom punctuated every event of my life and made even the worst crises bearable.

When I was 37, with three young daughters, my mom was diagnosed with leukemia. The foundation of my life shattered in a single phone call.

"What is it, mom, what did the doctor say?" I asked desperately, knowing she was calling with test results.

"Acute leukemia. I don't know what that means exactly, but Sweetie, it is not good," she replied in a low voice, full of caution and curiosity. She knew she was embarking on a frightening journey, with only uncertainty on the horizon.

The next three and a half years were consumed by test results, treatments, managing her medicines, her appointments, and my anxiety. I lived in a constant state of terror, fear for her pain, fear of her death. I did my best to take care of my mom, my dad, my kids, and my husband. I didn't follow the rule of self-care "put on your own oxygen mask first," and my health declined. Sleepless nights and anxiety-filled days, along with the pressure of trying to take care of everyone, overwhelmed me and I was physically and emotionally wasted.

After surviving three and a half dreadful treatment years which included chemotherapy, radiation, and two bone marrow transplants, my mom's cancer returned. Her doctors informed us that treatment options were exhausted. My mom received the news with sadness and dignity. Even in her last days in hospice care, she was still sharing wisdom.

After her final doctor's appointment, my aunt laid down next to my mom and said, "There's always hope, right Lottie?" "Until there isn't," my mom replied. She had accepted what was to come, but she was the only one who did.

Shortly before she died, I held her in my arms and begged her not to leave me. She placed her no longer beautifully manicured hand onto my chest and told me in a whisper, "I will always be here in your heart."

She knew she was dying, but she never stopped reminding me what was important in life. She knew that the power to endure challenges came from focusing on gratitude and joy.

"Go out and enjoy this beautiful day, Michelle, stop sitting in here with me being sad. Go find some joy and come back and tell me about it. Life is for the living!" she commanded weakly. I tried, but my mind and heart never really left her bedroom, except when I managed to make it to a yoga class.

Through those heartbreaking years, I had one health-supporting respite: my twice-weekly yoga classes. My teacher, Jim, would arrive at every class with a huge smile on his face and make jokes while he challenged our bodies, minds, and hearts to connect and align. For that blessed hour and fifteen minutes, while I felt challenge and pain, I was encouraged to hold steady and breathe through.

"Yoga helps you become comfortable with discomfort and thereby increases strength and resilience," Jim would say.

Yoga led me to develop strength, flexibility, and balance, within and beyond my physical body. As I extended into poses that required so much more than proper placement of my body parts, I began to feel physical, energetic, and spiritual alignment.

Frequently, I spent the last minutes of class crying silently in Savasana, the rest pose that completes every yoga practice. Yoga moved physical and emotional energy that was stuck in my body. Like the cracking of an iceberg, everything I had frozen and tried to hide away came crashing apart in the heat of the poses. I would hold on until the end of class, then, during rest, it all released, flowing out my eyes and sometimes causing my whole body to shake. Savasana was the most difficult pose for me. It was agonizing holding still while my thoughts and feelings churned.

Jim was very supportive, "Whatever comes out in Savasana, just go with it, crying, laughing, physical pain, thoughts, whatever happens, just keep breathing. You will find your strength in the silence."

While I grieved the loss of my mother, I could not accept that she was truly gone. She was my connection to the divine; I was angry and hopelessly lost without her presence. I needed her. There wasn't a moment of my life untouched by yearning for her guidance and love.

"Mom, you told me you would always be here!" I hissed quietly in frustration my first time back in synagogue shortly after her death. In the beautiful sanctuary where I grew up in Judaism, all I felt was her absence.

I lowered my head and sobbed silently, "Mom I need you; I can't do anything without you!" Watching my tears fall onto my hands, I focused on the beautiful ring of my mother's that I had been wearing since her death. It was yellow gold and shaped like a crown with a diamond plopped in the middle.

As I blinked away my tears, desperate for a connection with her, something shifted. I saw my hands, but I saw her hands. I closed my eyes and thought, *"Her hands are here, she isn't really gone."* I leaned into the feeling of her, my mother's presence was there. She could still support and comfort me. I breathed deeply into the imagined essence of her tuberose-scented perfume.

I could hear her words echoing through the space between us, "You can be anything you want, Michelle, you already have everything you need inside." In that moment, I experienced a greater sense of relief and love than I had since her diagnosis. I was still connected to her; she was still there, in my heart, in my mind, in the wisdom of the divine. I grasped at her, at that feeling, but it was fleeting.

I still felt powerless without her, still reaching for my mother to connect me to the divine. I was still a long way from understanding that everything I needed, the power of the divine, was inside me.

As I began to emerge from the trauma of my mother's death, I sought a deeper understanding of the meaning of life and death, and greater resilience to life's challenges. I knew yoga was a healing path, so to deepen my practice, I studied to become a yoga instructor.

Yoga teacher training taught me so much about myself. The physical practice was challenging, but the introspection required to apply yoga history and philosophy to my life was an even greater challenge. Looking inward only clarified how disconnected I was from my true nature.

When practiced diligently, yoga is a path to wholeness, healing, and union with the divine. I was so wrapped up in pain and grief, however, I had no ability to practice diligently. I had a vague understanding that living a yogic lifestyle could relieve my suffering and help me heal, but in my sorrow, I was unable to integrate those teachings into my life. Shame overwhelmed me because I was unable to gracefully recover from losing my mom. I hated myself. I numbed my pain with alcohol and prescription medications and other poor health choices.

The next years were spent slowly growing my yoga practice but suffering in my personal life. My marriage crumbled and I found myself divorced with three adolescent girls. I was consumed by taking care of my children and studying, but I was suffering deeply.

Seeking a more expansive understanding of yoga, I began training to be a yoga therapist. I was determined to learn how to help others, but I was still not attending to the personal care I needed to thrive. I didn't realize that looking only outward, I would never build the foundation of self-care I needed to be whole. I was not living what I was learning. Without loving and caring deeply for myself, I was incapable of truly loving anyone, including the divine spark inside me. I had forgotten my mother's teachings and Glinda's words.

Then I met Glen. Finally, I found the magic wizard who made my world perfect. He and I were like opposite poles of a magnet, drawn together with an inexplicable force; we fell immediately and deeply in love. I'm sure, when we met, the Earth tilted just a bit on its axis. With a wide-open heart, I let him lovingly pick up each piece of my shattered life and put them together to make me whole. He was strong, a trained fighter. I felt protected and at ease. Nothing bad could happen to me as long as I had his arms around me.

"Michelle, what took you so long to find me?" Glen asked me playfully four days after our first date. "I want you; I want to be with you always; I want to keep a smile on your face and never let anything hurt you again." I felt like I had fallen into a waking dream. He was so handsome, smart, funny, energetic and intense. When that intensity was focused on me, it made me feel invincible.

Could this man be for real? I thought. On that fourth day, I asked him hundreds of questions, all the red-flag deal breaker kind of questions best saved for after you've been dating someone for at least six months. He answered every question with such clarity and confidence it was as if he had a playbook for my heart.

He proposed to me a week after we met. He explained, "We need to be married; we already waited too long to meet each other." After three months, during which he continued to propose daily, we married. We couldn't see any reason to wait; we belonged together because after all, two broken pieces make a perfect whole. My disconnection from the divine seemed to be unimportant now.

Within a week, our lives were hit by a tornado. One of my daughters moved out and my ex-husband filed a custody and support lawsuit. Over the next several months, most of my family and friends vacated my life because they could not accept the choices I had made.

Even though Glen and I had our powerful love for support, the stress of loss and uncertainty strained us to the breaking point. We started drinking more alcohol and using other substances to ease our pain. Of course, things got worse. Alcohol lowers resilience. In time, the temporary escape we found in these unhealthy soothing techniques only brought greater misery.

Sixteen months after we married, the pressure was so high that Glen became depressed and hopeless. He began talking about suicide. I was terrified and desperately searched for ways we could heal. We tried to turn things around, got counseling and had some sober days, but things continued to get worse. One night he lost his temper and became violent with me. He hit me just once, but the words that accompanied the attack hurt even more.

Late that night, tucked into a ball, crying and afraid on my roommate's couch, I had a moment of silence, and clarity came to me. I felt a strength and knowing flow through me, from a source I could not identify. My inner wisdom spoke. "You need peace; you need to heal." The next day, I called upon my mom, the divine, and every bit of strength I could gather. I asked Glen to move out. I could not live with a man I feared.

Ironically, throughout that traumatic time, I was teaching up to twenty group yoga classes and coaching clients. Although that number of classes can be exhausting to teach, work was a respite for me. When I was in the studio, I felt safe.

Teaching and coaching take a great deal of mental energy and presence, and the focus they required kept me grounded. Teaching was my sanctuary. Yoga was my strength.

Although we were now living separately, Glen and I touched base almost every day. He told me he was getting help, he told me he was sober, and that he loved me. He promised he would never hurt me or himself. He begged me to let him move back in, but I struggled to trust him, so I kept putting him off. I still feared him and knew he needed to do more work on himself, for himself, before I would feel safe with him again.

Six weeks after Glen moved out, he followed through with his threat of suicide.

I nearly drowned under the wave of grief and shame that followed. I took a leave from work and stopped teaching for months. But instead of finding relief or any path to healing during that time, I made terrible choices. My substance abuse reached an all-time high as I did anything I could to escape from the pain. Just as I had after my mom's death, I forgot that my connection to the divine within was the only thing I needed to heal.

As I became despondent and desperate for relief, I contemplated following Glen into death. Finally, one dark November day, the friend that introduced me to Glen came to visit. This visit was the divine intervention that I needed.

My friend took one look at me and knew I was in trouble. He held my shoulders and looked intently into my eyes, connecting with me in a way I had not connected to anyone in longer than I could recall.

"Are you trying to die?" He asked me frankly, "Do you think you are stronger than these substances?" His questions shocked me. "I am going to contact you every day and if within two weeks, you don't have this under control, I am going to put you in rehab." This was not an empty threat; it was a promise.

At first, I laughed at him. The irony of a yoga teacher, yoga therapist, and wellness coach needing rehab was absurd.

"But I'm all about health!" I said defensively, mocking myself.
Then I broke down sobbing and hung my head in shame. Somewhere deep inside I knew he was speaking the truth. My connection with him that night was the gift of my life.

I cut back on substances immediately. I began seeing a trauma therapist and started down the difficult path of learning to manage the PTSD I had developed after Glen's death. With her help, I learned to reconnect with my body, and I went through the difficult process of getting sober. It wasn't a quick or easy journey, but it was a life-saving one. Sobriety cleared the way to my connection with the divine, and with myself.

A year after Glen died, I attended a meditation retreat. It was during this retreat that I met myself, for the first time, with compassion. This retreat deepened my knowledge of Ayurveda, the yogic science of total health. I began to fully understand that we are not separate beings, that we are all connected to and part of the divine natural order.

I received a personal mantra (a short phrase repeated silently as an object of focus) and started daily mantra meditation. Sitting in silence, meditating with over 400 people in a ballroom sanctuary, I felt divine power pulsing through me. In this healing environment with daily yoga and meditation practices, I reconnected and began to remember my power.

"Everything you need is inside you; you have the power; you just have to learn it for yourself." I could hear this wisdom flowing through me during meditation. I finally discovered the unknown source was inside me! I needed to stay connected to this source. I knew it was the path to my heart's desire.

After nearly dying of grief and substance abuse, my deepest desire was to become fully healthy of mind, body, and soul. This required looking inward for my divine spark and learning to love and accept myself completely.

I studied to become an Ayurvedic instructor, bringing yoga's wisdom into my daily life. The foundation of daily yoga and Ayurvedic practices gave me the strength to look at the unwise choices I made in my life and the damage my choices did to my relationships and my health.

Practicing compassion, forgiveness, equanimity, and gratitude, I slowly processed my pain, guilt, and shame. I apologized to everyone I knew I had hurt and I made efforts to repair relationships that remained unresolved, particularly my relationship with myself.

Continuing my healing journey, I studied shame, along with grief and PTSD. I wanted to know everything I could to help myself and others. I joined grief groups, suicide loss groups, and I raised money for suicide prevention. When I felt strong enough, I began to volunteer as a peer mentor for other suicide widows. Supporting another through their journey, I found, was a powerful way to strengthen and heal.

My own yellow brick road scarred and scared me. I often regretted venturing so far from home. But without my journey, I would not have learned that a bottle, my lover's arms, and even my mother's presence cannot alleviate my suffering.

I now see the scars from my experiences through the lens of appreciation for my journey. I appreciate that each challenge I faced was an opportunity for growth and a deeper understanding of the power I had all along. I know that gratitude for what I have, and for the joy in every moment, is the key to living a fulfilling and joyful life. I know that even on my darkest, most anxious days I can find comfort, just like on my mother's lap, in my connection to the divine presence within me.

When I am quiet and listen deeply with a clear, sober mind and an open heart, I see life itself as a miracle. The power to make my life a joyful and inspiring journey is deep within me and I don't even need ruby slippers to access it! True healing begins with the awareness that we are whole, perfect little humans made by and of divine wisdom.

My mom knew this when she slipped those beautiful shiny red shoes onto my feet for the first time, "You can be anything you want to be, Sweetie. You already have everything you need inside of you." I always had the power; I just had to learn it for myself.

About Michelle Ann Collins

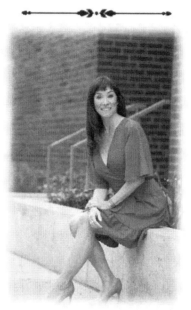

Michelle Ann Collins is an author, speaker, certified yoga therapist, and wellness coach who has taught yoga and mindfulness for over a decade. Michelle integrates the ancient practices of yoga and meditation combined with modern psychology and neuroscience to help her clients thrive. After suffering a series of heartbreaking losses, including the loss of her mother to cancer, her divorce, and losing her second husband to suicide, Michelle dove deeply into the healing studies of Ayurveda, yoga, meditation, and mindfulness. Through study and practice, she developed life-changing skills to survive, and ultimately thrive.

"Post-traumatic growth is possible and with the right coaching and support, no matter what challenges you face, you can live in vibrant health and joy."

—*Michelle Ann Collins*

www.inhabitjoy.com
Facebook: https://www.facebook.com/inhabitjoy
Instagram: michelleanncollins   Phone: (805)262-7806

INTEGRATION

Chapter 11
How A Catholic Girl Went to India and Found the Other Half of Her Soul

◆————————◆▶·◀◆————————◆

Anne Conley Ondrey

Mind vs Body

In ancient Greece, Plato postulated that the mind and the body are at odds and if we're smart, we'll select the mind as the superior side. Descartes later followed this up with "I think therefore I am" and the whole Western world marched forward into the realm of rational thought as our God Almighty. The Christian tradition neatly followed suit and the body was covered up, deprived of sex, sleep, starved and even flogged in an apparent effort to show the body that the mind is the boss. Like a frustrated parent of a wild two-year old, the Western mind clamped down hard on any requests from the body as messages from the devil incarnate.

Having grown up Catholic in the U.S., I knew a mild version of religious physical repression. In my late teens, I endured a stricter version during my time in the Pentecostal movement. It was the 1970s and in the New York City suburbs where I grew up, teens were either taking LSD or speaking in tongues. I was in the speaking in tongues group.

By my early twenties, I did an abrupt about face, went to college and played out a tame version of sex, pot, and rock and roll. Towards my thirties, I returned to the Catholic Church, which was easier now as a married woman with children. But there was dissonance still between my mind and my body and I didn't know exactly what it was or what to do about it.

Pre-Yoga

I'm born under the sign of Gemini and we're thought of as thinkers – not feelers. I'm a constant consumer of books, classes, podcasts, TED Talks, or really anything cognitive. But part of me knew all along that something was missing with all this thinking.

In my early 30s, I ran a small non-profit agency after completing my Masters in Social Work in Community Organization. It was hard work, raising money, leveraging resources, and cajoling anyone and everyone to lend a hand.

One day I was in my office and a woman asked to see me. She had received a free mammogram through our program at the local hospital. The nurse in charge of the clinic had warned me that one client had been very difficult and she suspected I'd be hearing from her. So my antenna went up as I realized this was probably that woman.

As she launched into her myriad of complaints about our free mammogram service, I began to feel an incredibly strange sensation welling up in my body. Even though she was talking, I stopped hearing her. All of my attention was focused on an almost frightening sensation that had started in my hips and was now moving up my spine like a snake, powerful and hot. All of a sudden, I realized I was on the verge of screaming at her to get out of my office. I awkwardly got her to leave while barely managing to repress the scream.

After it was over, all attention turned away from my body and returned back to my thinking mind. I reasoned I was overtired and my mind just dismissed the experience. But Yoga, India, and chanting were on my horizon.

Enter Yoga

"Where do you feel it in your body?" In my forties, this is what my Gestalt therapist would ask me when I was struggling with a difficult memory or thought. Truly I wanted to jump out of my chair and throttle her. I didn't want to *feel* the thought. I wanted to *think* the thought. But I did begin to try and I began to feel, even if it was just a little bit. And don't worry – I never throttled her. In fact, I can never thank her enough.

During those sessions, it came to me that I should really try yoga. My mother had done yoga in the 1960s and I had been curious about it. I finally found a class at a local Catholic convent that had a spirituality center. That class led to other classes, which led to yoga teacher training, which led to a complete job and life change.

Enter Chanting

I'd been teaching yoga for about five years and was taking yet another training when the instructor mentioned a trip to India. She said it wasn't a tour – it was a chanting pilgrimage. She'd been twice and was going again. I wrote the information down in my notebook, the way I write everything down in my notebook. But my mind was already creating roadblocks against the trip.

This same instructor then chanted a mantra (a repeated sacred word or phrase) that stopped me in my tracks. When she chanted it, I felt a huge shift in my body, like the way an 18-wheeler thuds when jake braking. I asked if she would provide me with a copy of the mantra and she did. It was a salutation to the Hindu deity Ganesha, who like all Hindu deities, represents an aspect of the one Divine God. Ganesha is the remover of obstacles, those things in our lives that we wish would go away but often produce great personal growth.

I returned home from the training and slowly and steadily learned the Ganesha mantra. When I shifted to silent meditation, the Indian pilgrimage would float right up into my consciousness. I dismissed the thought every time it came up, thinking the trip too expensive and, at three weeks, too long to be away. But the thought was so persistent that I finally looked the trip up online. It was less expensive than I thought. I mentioned it to my husband, thinking he'd nix the idea.

"I think you should go," he said, much to my surprise. "And I think you should go this year because you can." It seemed Ganesha was at work, removing obstacles and opening my path to India.

India: The Other Half of Our Soul

I signed up for the trip wondering what this would lead to in my life. Three months later, I emerged from a Lufthansa plane into Chennai, India, leaving behind the frozen North to dive into the warm South with its vibrant hues and pungent smells (some flowery and others fetid). We went to a hotel on the Bay of Bengal where we would rest up before heading by train seven hours West to the ashram, which would be our home base. Called Shantivanam (Forest of Peace), the ashram, like many of South India's sacred spaces, is located along the banks of the Cauvery River.

The pilgrimage was led by Russill Paul, author of *The Yoga of Sound: Tapping the Hidden Power of Music and Chant*. Paul has been leading the pilgrimage with his wife, Asha, for 20 years. It's a journey, he says, to find the other half of our soul – the Eastern half – the part that Plato, Descartes and the Western church conveniently cut out. We would be chanting ancient mantras and visiting Hindu temples so old that they were built towards the beginning of the Common Era.

I didn't learn a lot about the ashram before going but once there I realized it was founded by two Catholic priests. Their goal was to integrate the monasticism of sixth-century St. Benedict, known as the Father of Western monasticism, with the spirituality of a Hindu ashram, or the other half of the soul. This became known as the Christian Ashram Movement. I was partly amused, due to my Catholic

136

heritage, as well as curious, intrigued, and a little apprehensive about the shifts that I sensed were ahead for me.

Starting to Practice

The initiation ceremony at the ashram took place at night in the meditation hall. As with all things Indian, the event was a visual extravaganza – piles of bright yellow flowers strewn in the center of our circle scattered with deep red flower petals amidst glowing candles. Each of us received a saffron scarf to wear as the universal Eastern sign that we were seekers of God. We also received a set of mala beads to use for chanting (I noticed that a mala has 108 beads while a Catholic rosary has exactly half that amount at 54 beads).

As we began to chant together, the group took on a rhythmic pulse like the wheels of a train starting slowly and then picking up speed. I felt a churning inside of me, a sensation I had experienced the very first time I'd ever chanted. It was during a yoga class several years prior and the teacher had put on a CD for us to chant along with. I was seated on the floor with my legs crossed and as I started to chant, my torso began to slowly circle, quite independent of my mind – just like the episode in my office with the complaining woman. The initiation of this movement came completely from my body as I chanted and again took me by complete surprise.

Practice, Practice, Practice

At the ashram, we chanted together for several hours each day, often slowly circling as we chanted. One day about a week into the trip, when the novelty was beginning to wear off, I wasn't feeling any of those powerful sensations. I felt bored and I aimlessly looked around at the ashram as I chanted and circled thinking "there's that cow again" or "there's that hut again" round and round and round. But suddenly I realized there was a distinction between the chattering in my mind and the slow, steady pulse of the chant as it resonated through my body. I also realized that these were two different things! These were two separate streams of experience and I could choose to observe the thinking but sink into the inner heartbeat of the chant. In Catholicism, I could never find this inner heartbeat when saying prayers or the rosary. There were just a lot of words about God in my head but not this primal vibration inside my body.

Spidey Sense

Occasionally, we'd have sessions at night. One was in the moonlight on the banks of the Cauvery and, except for a few bugs, was soft and dreamy. But on another night, we were in the meditation hall and it was torturous. I was convinced a spider had landed on the top of my head and had released an army of baby spiders who were crawling down my scalp. It was all I could do to not run out of the hall screaming.

When the session finally ended, I asked a friend to look at my head with a flashlight to check for spiders. But there weren't any there. I had no idea what was happening to me but my skin itched for a shower with hot water to wash off whatever had come to the surface. We didn't have hot water at the ashram but we could ask ashram staff for special requests. I was able to procure a bucket of hot water from the kitchen. It was around nine and by then most everyone at the ashram was asleep. Combining the blessedly hot water from the bucket with the cold water from the shower spigot, I felt I was washing off layers of sadness and pain that had weighed down my spirit, what we call samskaras in yoga. It felt like a true baptism, unlike my infant baptism, and I was baptizing myself. I radiated a newness, and the Western half of my soul, the rational, thinking, logical part that I grew up with, couldn't explain it.

In *The Yoga of Sound*, Paul explains how unpleasant sounds or "noise pollution" negatively affect our bodies. Physics tells us that our bodies and everything in them vibrate. Mantras work with these vibrations and are the language of yoga, like mathematics is the language of science. For generations, yogic mantras have been selected to promote an individual's wellbeing. As apparently happened in my body that night, the mantra dissolved stuck energy and opened the flow within what yoga calls our subtle body. Our subtle body coexists with our physical body and has its own nervous system composed of channels called nadis. Much like meridians in Chinese medicine, when our energy flows smoothly along these nadis, we expand and thrive.

Visiting the Indian Temples

To prepare for our first temple visit, we put on our saffron scarves and marked our foreheads with holy ash (not just on Ash Wednesday as in the West). Once inside the temple, we circumambulated around the sacred space, a carefully designed and mathematically-organized grid. It was at this point that I felt another physical response not under my conscious control: pressure all around my throat like a tiny turtleneck squeezing my neck. It was uncomfortable but it felt like a response to awe, perhaps the way Moses felt at the burning bush. Later we watched a ritual pooja (Hindu worship ceremony) completed by a Swami who adorned Hindu's sacred lingam and yoni. The lingam is a phallus-shaped statue representing the Divine Masculine energy of Shiva and it rests in the yoni, an oval-stone base representing the Divine Feminine energy of Shakti. The Swami chanted mantras in a sequence as he poured water, honey, bananas, milk, and flowers over the lingam. One of the women in our group was so aroused by the physicality and sensuality of the pooja that when she returned to the ashram, she called her partner in the U.S. to have phone sex!

At another temple, called the Rock Fort, we ascended 344 steps to a pooja for Ganesha, chanting as we climbed. The rock of this temple is said to be 3.8 billion years old. The force of the chanting and the swami raising a large temple lamp called a diyas above our heads dropped me into an altered state. I felt deeply satisfied like I'd been submerged in a pool of cool water on a scorching day. This light, representing in Hinduism the Divine presence itself, felt vast and ancient but current and palpable. It didn't matter that our group was Caucasian from the U.S. and that the other devotees were Southeast Asian. All differences melted away in a universality that I'd never felt when consuming the eucharist at a Catholic Mass. These visually and sonically rich poojas reached down into my gut in an instinctual way – no thinking involved. One can see how the sexually-repressed English colonizers viewed these practices as pagan and even dangerous as they arouse our primal and sensual selves.

The Catholicism I was raised with had small elements of this richness. Although I played my guitar at folk mass in the gym during the 1960s, it was in our Gothic revival church where I felt the hush, mystery, and reverence of the Divine that I later found so deeply in India. I could get lost looking up at the rib-vaulted ceiling and at the pendant chandeliers suspended on their long, metal chains; I felt enveloped in the rays of red and blue light streaming through the stained-glass windows. I even felt the sanctity of the cave-like confessionals in the back of the church. But the services emphasized purity and prayers and my body felt ignored and repressed.

Most Catholics are familiar with instructions against self-pleasuring. Even the roots of the word masturbation are negative: manus comes from hand and turbare from to disturb. The idea that exploring our bodies with our God-given hands is wrong is a mental construct created by our fear bodies for supposed protection. Locking my body away from my experience, as I had been taught in my childhood religion, created a disconnect that was now being healed.

Dreamy Consciousness

After a profoundly spiritual day trip to an ashram run by Hindu nuns (yoginis) where we witnessed a five-hour homa or fire pooja, I lay down to sleep with the chant of Om

Namah Shivaya (Universal Consciousness is One) running on a loop in my head. I lapsed into a vivid dream where I am a very small but brilliant white light in a sea of infinite blackness. There are an endless number of other small, brilliant lights. The peace was all encompassing, truly the peace that passeth all understanding; the rhythm was collectively flawless as we flowed like an enormous unit. The span of the lights and the darkness was limitless, the sense of a vast, ultimate power humbling, showing me the truth that I am truly a small speck – albeit an important speck – in a massive, collective whole. As I started to awaken, I had that odd feeling of not knowing where I was except this time, I didn't know who I was. My ego and personality had vanished, just as all spiritual practices invite us to do. When I awoke, I wanted to go back to that dream place of undulating, unified peace. I was disappointed to find myself back in my body that now felt claustrophobic, like being jammed between the walls of a narrow cave. In a way, I've wanted to go back to that dream ever since.

Coming Home

I'd love to tell you my coming home went smoothly, but it didn't. I returned to gray, cold Northeast Ohio from sunny, balmy South India. By June, I was ill, exhausted, losing weight and having abdominal pain. Weeks of tests discovered no diagnosis other than that my immune system was sluggish. I began to think of it as a kind of failure to thrive. I would cry when I thought about India and I had a deep ache for life at the ashram with its cadence of calm, which was so different from my punishing work schedule in the U.S. So I took a month off and rested. I returned to daily chanting, using a CD I had brought home from the ashram. Slowly, my health returned.

In the 1960s, a similar malady affected a group of French, Benedictine monks when they replaced chanting many hours each day in Gregorian Chant with spoken prayers in their native language. The change, initiated to modernize the church in response to the Second Vatican Council, created illness. Following a lifetime of chanting, many monks lay listless in their cells. No one knew what was wrong with them but a doctor recommended they return to chanting. Within nine months, all were restored to full health. Reestablishing their chanting practice reconnected them with their internal rhythm and with the subtle frequencies humming through the channels of their bodies.

Chanting quite literally changes our bodies. I know because it changed mine. At times, chanting is profound; other times, it's ecstatic. Sometimes, it's just repetitive. But the key for me is to chant daily, regardless of my mood, which is changeable like the weather.

The word yoga means to yoke ourselves to something bigger than ourselves so we surrender our ego. When we chant, we do this. We connect ourselves with this ancient, sonic-stream of sound that vibrates within all the cells of our bodies. It's a mystery that makes no sense to the rational mind of the West. But it makes perfect sense to the intuitive, other half of our souls, for which I am eternally grateful.

About Anne Conley Ondrey

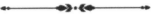

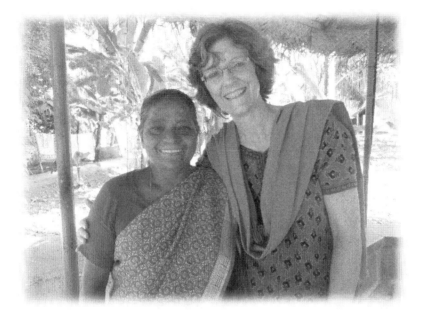

(Anne with a Catholic nun and social worker from the nearby village.)

Anne Conley Ondrey has a BA from Brown University and a Masters in Social Work from the University of Pittsburgh. She has enjoyed careers as a journalist, social worker and yoga instructor. She is a registered yoga instructor, yoga therapist and a Reiki Master specializing in anatomy, restorative yoga and chair yoga. She is deeply grateful to her many teachers as well as to her students for their instruction and compassion. A native New Yorker, she now lives outside of Cleveland, OH, with her husband, Thomas, and delights in her two grown children, son-in-law and two grandchildren.

You can visit her website at
www.theyogapathonline.com

Chapter 12
A Flow of Grace
From Effort to Ease

Claire M Zovko

When I reflect back on my upbringing, I think of a household with a lot of people, with a lot of action, and a lot of needs that needed to be met. My two parents raised me in the Seattle, Washington area as the youngest of eight children.

I loved being around all of my siblings. My brother is the closest sibling in age so I tagged along with him. Whatever my brother did, I did. Building treehouses, rollerblading, or playing sports. As a young kid, adventure always excited me.

I recall a natural competition element and a lot of doing throughout childhood. From birth through junior high, it felt like a competition for time with my parents or even competing for basic necessities, or for the money available in the household to meet needs.

One specific occasion that impacted me immensely occurred on Christmas Day. All day we enjoyed a wonderful holiday together as a big family. That night, my siblings decided to go see a movie that happened to be PG-13. As a ten-year-old, the invitation to the movie did not extend to me. After having this amazing holiday together, they all said, "We are off to the movies!"

I was left at home. I remember feeling sad and feeling lonely. At that age, I took it personally. My mind could not fully process why they left me out. For me, though the age factor is out of my control, it really felt unfair. Subconsciously it felt that I was not good enough to be able to go with them. It really bothered me. It felt horrible to be left out.

From the home environment and especially after that situation, a desire to prove myself became present. I yearned to show that I was good enough through a wide variety of outlets, so I would not be left behind again. I played numerous sports and I would seek to be very successful at them. Also, with academics, I wanted to be very successful to validate myself, and not be left out.

When I got to high school, the family dynamics shifted. Now all of my siblings were in college or beyond. They all moved out and left the house to live their lives. I experienced home life as an only child. Compared with growing up, the contrast felt like night and day. For the first time, I experienced my parents always being available. I no longer had to compete for their time. Now there were ample resources for the basic things that I needed.

My parents had been strict with some of my other siblings. Yet, by the time I got to high school, they did not have the energy or interest to regulate every single aspect of my life. They were laid back and just trusted me. As my focus remained committed to sports and academics, they allowed me the freedom and space to just BE and explore during that time.

In high school, athletics were the cornerstone of my experience. I played a different sport every season. I also enjoyed academics as it came naturally to me. Through sports and academics, it validated me, which made that time a pleasant experience. The issues of self-worth were mending but still buried deep beneath the surface.

Basketball took predominance over all sports in my life through college. I finished my senior year of college and the basketball season came to an end. This time in life felt unique and unfamiliar as I pondered the question—"Who am I?" Previously, I always defined myself as an athlete, a basketball player. I tied everything around that identity, and the identity ended.

This unknown place felt like an identity crisis of sorts. In this confusing time, I serendipitously stumbled across yoga. One day while visiting my aunt, she invited me to a join her for yoga class. I did not know the first thing about yoga but I excitedly said, "Yes!" I took my first yoga class and life would never be the same. The yoga journey started rolling from there.

When I first started, I practiced a style called Bikram Yoga that opened my eyes to deeper layers of physicality. Through this practice, I began to feel my body in new ways. To not only be challenged but be challenged by myself; challenged by my own bodyweight. I previously relied on external things such as weights to be challenged. This was different. It provided me the opportunity to discover new aspects of myself.

The yoga demanded extreme focus and intention of every detail in each moment. A small shift of awareness impacted the experience in the pose. Even though the athletics gave me strength, I realized quickly that I lacked flexibility. Within I felt a huge imbalance where I did not have the flexibility to support the strength in my body. Class by class, the yoga practice started to open me physically.

I practiced that style of yoga for seven years with dedication to the practice. Then, I came to a point where I had a realization and thought, "What I am doing in the yoga room is exactly what I am doing in my life. Even though I am in the yoga room and it is beautiful, I am still hard on myself. I am still judging myself. I am still competing. I am still not good enough. I am in a hot room kicking my own ass with a bunch of other people. It is the same thing that I have always done, but now it is in a new environment."

After that awakening, I experienced my first Vinyasa Yoga class. For the first time, I started to experience the feeling and sensation of postures being connected, the free flow of a class, and a variety of sequences. For the first time, I moved my body in such a graceful and flowing way. Again, my eyes were opened wide. "Wow, where have I been?" I really lacked fluidity in my way of being up until that point. Until I allowed myself to move in a way with more freedom and grace, rigidity had been my natural state.

My chosen profession brought forward another pivotal moment. I attended law school, still rigid and overachieving. When I finished law school, I faced another turning point. Now I needed to decide, am I going to stay in Florida where I went to law school? Am I going to move back home where it is comfortable? Or am I going to find a new city and have a new life adventure? I could no longer use education as a crutch to hold on to certainty in life.

The unknown again is sitting right in front of me. In this moment, it feels scary with no direction. I am wondering, "What am I going to do? There is no basketball. There is no school anymore." From the yoga practice, even though that moment brought up a lot of fear, I felt an openness to it, a flow to it. I took a moment to pause and say, "If I really see what has unfolded, living in Miami for the last three years, a natural, organic network has set itself up. Why would I run away from this?" I feel the yoga practice gave me the courage to stay in Miami and trust a greater plan. Now 15 years later, I am still here.

The yoga journey continued to grow and expand. Now I finished law school, which challenged me massively academically. I felt that, "If I can complete law school, I can do anything at this point." That is when I felt called in my heart to take yoga teacher training. Even though I did not have the intention to become a yoga teacher, the call to deepen my practice inspired me to take the leap.

After the teacher training, I could feel the beginning of a new way of being and living. It felt like the first step on the evolutionary path of yoga that I felt so drawn to.

I began to teach yoga for a couple of years, and I really loved it. I loved sharing with people the transformational tools that I experienced through the practice. Sharing the yoga felt organic. I could not help but share. After a couple years of teaching yoga once a week, I got to a point where I felt I hit a plateau and said the same things over and over again. I felt I needed to learn more.

In Miami, I took another yoga teacher training at a local studio to go deeper. This particular training included a plethora of different yoga styles with the top teachers of those unique styles in South Florida. I became exposed to Kundalini, Iyengar, Anusara, prenatal, kids yoga—all these different aspects that I had no clue about. Again, I felt an expansion of how I experienced the yoga practice and life.

When I finished that training, I started teaching right away at the local studio. At that point, I taught four classes a week, and shared the practices as much as I could while practicing law daily.

A living yoga master, Anand Mehrotra, came from India to visit the United States. While in the States, he held a weekend experience at the studio that I taught at. He shared multiple wisdom talks and a journey that were beyond anything that I had ever experienced before.

After meeting him, the whole course of my life changed. This moment of grace shifted everything though I did not know it at the time. In the wisdom talk, I remember he spoke about quantum leaps beyond my state of consciousness. I did not even understand what he discussed, yet my soul cheered and said, "Truth! Truth!" Everything that he said, my soul agreed with, even though my conscious mind thought, "I do not even know what is happening right now."

I had never felt this way in the presence of any human being. A deep feeling of pure truth on a cellular level. In that moment, I knew I had to study further with him. Two years later, I went to India and took my 300-hour teacher training with him. This is where I learned a comprehensive daily meditation technique.

For about nine years, I had practiced as a lawyer with a few boutique law firms. Little by little, the practice of law started fading away and the yoga started exponentially growing. Eventually, the flow of grace brought me into teaching law at the University of Miami and the practice of law became less and less.

At that time, I could keep the law and yoga separate. I had a legal life and then I had a yoga life. I did not mix them too much—the lawyers I worked with probably did not know that I taught yoga. For a long time, the yoga students did not know that I practiced law. People really did not know because I lived my life with two silos and kept them compartmentalized. Once I started seeing these two aspects of myself not in opposition but as complementary, then I became fully open about all of it. I stopped hiding and started showing up fully.

I met Anand in 2014. I continue to study with him at Sattva Yoga Academy and have made frequent pilgrimages to Rishikesh, India to continue to learn the ancient wisdom. As I kept exploring the practice of yoga, every step on this path felt so natural and guided.

For me, the meditation practice changed the way that I experienced life. For a long time, I wanted to meditate, but I could not sit still for more than a minute or two. I learned the comprehensive technique and started practicing it daily. Meditation brought me immense peace, clarity, and stillness, which felt unfamiliar. Coming from my background of so much doing and achieving in the past, meditation felt like the exact opposite. Previously I kept moving to avoid having to feel what lingered under the surface and the lack of self-worth. Now, by having meditation, it gave me time and space to experience myself outside of the things that I do. I began to be with myself and really understand and explore myself like I have never done before.

When that first training in India concluded, the opportunity to ride on the back of a motorcycle presented itself. Without thinking too much, I said "Yes!" Before this moment, motorcycles did not interest or appeal to me. In fact, I thought motorcycles were scary and even dangerous.

As a motorcycle passenger, I quickly started to experience immense bliss, connection, and unity. I felt deeply connected to myself, the driver, the surroundings and life itself. We were one as we weaved through the Himalayan winding roads and rural communities.

At the end of the day, I hopped off the bike in pure joy. I thought, "Wow, if this experience is so powerful riding on the back of the bike, I can only imagine how powerful it is being in the driver's seat."

When I returned home stateside, I enrolled in a riding course, got my motorcycle endorsement, and I took up motorcycle riding. I became inspired to learn because Anand guides a spiritual journey where he takes bikers through the Himalayas. So I started practicing this new undertaking, and immediately signed up for the 2018 motorcycle journey.

Motorcycles were new to me, and I had only ridden a handful of times before riding in India. Our group consisted of Anand, 20 riders, 13 passengers, two mechanics, and three support staff. We embarked on a three-week journey through the Himalayas. The journey took us to what is known as "The Highest Pass", Khardung La. The peak is at 18,379 feet and one of the highest motorable roads in the world.

It is still surreal to me. We rode on these roads that barely looked like roads. We rode through all possible terrains and all possible weather conditions. But really, the journey went beyond the act of riding. We had the chance to access our Highest Self. Throughout the experience, my stuff came up, along with everyone else's. We had to go through our issues to be able to access our hidden potentiality. The depth of the journey allowed me to face the deepest parts of myself that I avoided for so long. Through the challenges and opposition, it opened my eyes to see life in a whole new way.

The turning point of the journey for me happened to be on the second day of riding. Again, I am a new rider, and I have never ridden 12-14 hours a day before or even more than a couple of hours. On that day, somewhere in the Himalayas, in the middle of nowhere, after riding eight hours, I hit my breaking point. We were stuck in standstill traffic in 100-something degree weather with the sun shining right on us. I felt hungry. I felt physically sore and exhausted. I felt emotionally exhausted. I felt socially exhausted. I had all the full riding gear on, and I sweated profusely while internally feeling like I would explode. I just could not do it anymore.

I told the rider next to me, "I can't do this. I am done. This is just too crazy." Right away he jumped off his motorcycle and ran to a car with our support team. The mechanic came right out and jumped on my bike, so I could get off the bike immediately. My headspace did not allow me to be on that bike one minute longer. I jumped into the support vehicle and I broke down in tears. I struggled. I felt frustration and anger at myself. I asked myself over and over, "Why can't I keep up? How is everyone else able to do this, but I am not?" Again, the self-worth issue arose. Again, I identified myself by what I could or could not do.

For the next two hours until we got to the peak that evening, I had a pity party with myself in shambles. We got to the top and finally stopped for lunch at 5pm. I got out of the car and ran into Anand right away. He said, "Claire, are you okay?" I felt so much anger and frustration in that moment, I just said, "NO! I am not okay!" and I stomped off. I do not ever show up like that so this moment definitely stuck out as odd. I went off to be by myself. I broke down in tears. I felt this huge breaking point where I could not keep it together any longer.

Anand came by to check in, and he asked, "What's going on?" I shared with him the experience. Then he said to me, "Claire, do you see the grace? In the moment that you needed support, your fellow rider immediately helped you. The mechanic jumped right out and rode your bike. A support car picked you up. You had A/C in the middle of the Himalayas and you were carried to the top with ease." He emphasized, "Do you see the grace? Focus on the grace. See the grace."

In that moment, my consciousness expanded. I realized and saw the egoic pattern of feeling a lack of self-worth. I thought, "Look where I am at right now. Never in a million years could I have guessed I would be in the Himalayas on a mountain top riding a motorcycle with dear soul family. *How did I get here?* Grace is what truly surrounded me in that moment." Until he pointed it out, I did not see it. That moment of seeing and feeling the omnipotent grace that is will always stick with me.

From this experience, I now see the relevance of tearing down things that the ego created so that there is space for Divine purpose, Divine gifts, and Divine alignment to flow through one's life. It is really a shift from struggle to flow, and from effort to ease.

The yoga is no longer something that I do. The yoga is a way of being and it is something that I love to practice every day. I hold it close to my heart. I am now open to the Divine plan. I continue to let go daily of Claire's plan, and open more and more to the Divine plan. Everything in nature grows and evolves. That is what I seek to be in alignment with and stay in alignment with—to continue to grow and evolve.

Through these life experiences, I feel the capacity to understand others has grown. Previously, I felt that I could only understand people like me, but now, from the practice and expansion, it is easier to see others as they are.

Now when I teach at the University, I start every class with what I call a 'mindful minute.' It is essentially a guided meditation where we tune into the moment before we dig into the legal material. I can no longer be without the yoga in all aspects of life. The separation I used to experience is now deeply felt as interconnection.

I feel more fluid than ever and that things beyond me are happening through me. There is more love. There is more appreciation. There is more grace. There is more seeing myself. There is more seeing others for who they are. There is more compassion. There is more forgiveness. A lot of those things were lacking pre-yoga.

When I reflect back on the yoga path, it really took me to the highest part of the world and endless doing to realize to be in the grace that has been along the path the whole time. In all of the busyness, I ran right by it. *How am I experiencing my life now? How has the yoga impacted me and others?* It is all just grace. A beautiful flow of grace.

To experience a sense of grace and ease within, I recommend a simple technique called Balanced Breath. Simply track your breath's four parts—the inhale, a pause, the exhale, and a pause at the bottom. Take each part to an internal count of four. Inhale for a count of four, hold your breath for four, exhale for four, hold your breath for four. This simple practice four minutes a day can cultivate a shift from effort to ease.

About Claire M Zovko, Esq., E-RYT

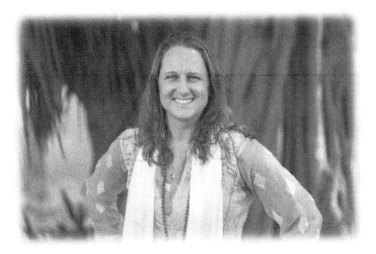

Claire M Zovko, Esq., E-RYT is a pioneer in conscious living, visionary, evolutionary thought leader, and entrepreneur. She is the founder of Lighthouse Yoga & Wellness and the *Light on Being* podcast. As a natural teacher, she has guided hundreds of students to awaken their potential, embody Divine purpose, and live life fully. Claire studied the Yog Vedantic lineage through many pilgrimages to Rishikesh, India at Sattva Yoga Academy. As a Sattva Yoga & Meditation Master Teacher and Jyotishi, she shares Kriya Yoga, meditation initiations, Dasha Mahavidya Goddess Sadhana, and Vedic Astrology readings. Her innate ability to clearly communicate brings the sacred teachings forward in a simple way. On her spiritual journey, she traveled the world through over 40 countries, loves learning, and brings universal wisdom to students.

Lighthouse Yoga & Wellness
www.lighthouseyogawellness.com

Instagram @Clairez1111 @LightonBeing

SACRED FEMININE HEALING

Chapter 13
My Healing Hands:
A Skeptic Opens to the Miraculous

Hyla Hitchcox

A sneering voice, accompanied by a look of disgust at my gnarled fingers, came from a customer in the bagel shop: "You're not going to make my sandwich with those hands, are you?"

An amazed, grateful voice drifted up from a client on the massage table: "Are those really your hands, not heaters?" Both questions were asked about my hands, a decade apart. The first triggered shame, the second, confidence.

In between, I became a Healer, and the Healer's journey is a twisty road indeed.

What does it mean to heal, and to be a Healer? Healing is an ever-changing process, not a goal. Healing means growing and deepening into our true selves, which may or may not involve curing. It is possible to be dying and yet healed, to be cured and yet remain a stranger to one's self.

By first learning to heal one's self, the Healer can assume the role of a catalyst for growth, with the intention to heal others, and openness to, without expectation of, miracles.

Think about your hands, and the hands of your loved ones and ancestors. Hands hold, grasp, push, pull, and let go. Hands can hurt or heal others, and even hurt or heal ourselves. We learn about the world through touch, and we rely on healthy touch as an essential part of life. Babies, lacking touch, fail to thrive. Our hands and hearts are inextricably linked. The twists and turns of our lives are deeply influenced by our holding on and our letting go, literally and metaphorically. It is easy to take our hands for granted, until we cannot use them.

My mom's hands were arthritic and painful, but she did not let that stop her from doing what brought her joy: gardening. She was in the garden almost every day, nurturing her daylilies, vegetables, and fruit bushes. She also brought babies into the world. At her memorial, many attended whose grown children had been delivered into her welcoming hands.

My dad had strong hands that worked with wood and stone, metal and bone. He collected fossils, and even unearthed a mammoth tusk, that he kept in a closet. He built much of my childhood home, and maintained our cars. When my parents were in the midst of their divorce, he built a beautiful stone retaining wall to buttress one of my mom's flowerbeds, channeling his broken heart into creativity.

My parents, disillusioned by their high-pressure evangelical Christian roots, had joined the back-to-the-land movement before I was born, and raised me to question everything, be kind, and celebrate the wonder of the natural world. They both had a deep connection to the earth, the stars, and the seasons. They loved to dig in the soil, turning the compost to nurture our burgeoning organic gardens. Every year, we would venture into the woods to gather decomposing leaves to add to the garden. We picked wild berries and identified birds by sight and song. My dad studied geology and taught me about fossils and rocks and minerals.

Some of my earliest memories are of my dad pointing out constellations on our nightly walks around the lake, as I lay back in my stroller, gazing at the sky: Cassiopeia, Orion, The Pleiades and the wondrous swath of the Milky Way. I learned about the phases of the moon, and the cycles of the seasons as my Dad shared his scientific musings laced with wonder. This sparked in me a deep, abiding connection to nature.

I was labeled "gifted" at age six, which, as the years passed, felt increasingly more like an expectation to live up to than a gift. Though I was a precocious reader, and had "book smarts", I had very little confidence in myself, and froze in the face of any decision, even something as simple as choosing what to eat.

I was painfully shy. Even as a senior in high school, I was voted "most shy", and several classmates wrote in my yearbook: "I wish I could have gotten to know you if you weren't so shy." Ouch. But, I wonder, would they really have gotten to know me? I hardly knew myself. I could ace a test, but I genuinely could not have told you what my own opinions were.

I was intimidated by my dad's overbearing presence. He knew what his opinions were, and would express them to anyone. He seemed oblivious to personal boundaries. Years of counseling and the outside perspective of friends opened my eyes to the emotional and indirect sexual abuse that I experienced. My dad could justify anything, usually in the interest of education, including exposing himself to me when I was nine.

When I was fourteen, and away at camp, my dad tore down my room, leaving me without privacy just as I was entering puberty. A roof leak was the justification, but I was without a private space for the next 3 years. A year later, when I came home from school early to find him, naked, on the living room couch that doubled as my bed, he claimed it was common space, not "my bed". However, that couch was the only personal space I had in the house. It would be two more years until he built me a new room. Having so little privacy in those formative years was deeply challenging.

My mom was an accomplished labor and delivery nurse, and later a much loved teacher to the next generation of nurses. But at home, she was the passive counterpoint to my dad's domineering personality. If asked about their marriage, she summed it up with "Well, I made my bed, and now I have to lie in it." She preferred to retreat to her garden, and rarely stepped in when my dad was teasing me like an ornery big brother. When I asked her many years later why she didn't step in more often, she apologized and said my dad was upset when she "sided against him", saying they should be "a united front", when dealing with me, their only child, as if I was the enemy.

Two years before the loss of my room, and my privacy, my heart and mind had been deeply traumatized when I witnessed a suicide. After school one day, my friend and I saw Lee, the fifteen-year-old brother of another friend, sitting in a bus shelter. Coming closer to say hello, we saw that he had a rifle. He asked us to go away. When we returned a little while later, he was lying on the ground, alive, but bleeding profusely, having shot himself in the chest. Someone had called 911 and the sirens filled the air. (It would be many years before the sound of sirens no longer triggered a panic attack in me.) As he lay there, he poked his finger at the wound, repeating over and over "Let me die." We later found out that Lee had died that night at the hospital.

I didn't even begin to feel, let alone start to process Lee's suicide until I was in high school. What surfaced was guilt, wondering if I could have done something, fear, wondering if he might have shot us, and anger, as I wondered how he could be selfish enough to take his own life.

High school is not an easy time for many people, and I was no exception. My family dynamic and the trauma had built up to the point of combustion, but I was shy and passive and it all turned inward. I was a good student, but my inner world was fraught with anxiety: panic attacks and insomnia plagued me most nights.

Eczema appeared on my hands. I remembered having small patches of it on the backs of my knees as a small child, but it had been gone for years. This time, it was relentless: an itch that made me want to tear my skin, peaking at night and worsening as I got older. Self-conscious, I hid my hands in my pockets when I could, avoiding the inevitable stares.

My hands were always itchy, often cracked and swollen, sometimes bleeding or weeping, with a mosaic of bandages over the deepest fissures. Rubbing them against fabric or running hot water over them eased the itch briefly, but caused more swelling, cracking, and bleeding. I tried salves and ointments, acupuncture, and steroid creams. It would nearly go away, and then "the itch that rashes" would begin again in a never-ending cycle.

In college, my eczema continued to worsen, and I searched for ways to ease my anxiety. I explored yoga, meditation, and dance. I loved doing yoga, and yet I felt embarrassed, blocked, and was unable to bring myself to make "prayer hands" or say "Namaste". I wanted to be calm and free from anxiety and itching and pain, but I just couldn't allow myself to let go of judgment and my own victim mentality. They seemed so fake to me, those smiling, open hearted, "Namaste"-ing people, but really I was jealous. I allowed myself to consider that maybe they really meant it. And if so, I wondered, what was their secret?

Emotional breakthroughs emerged as time passed. One day, I was doing a headstand when suddenly, out of the blue, it was as if my soul was turned upside down: the dam broke, and out poured a river of tears: concentrated years of pain, anger, guilt, grief, and exhaustion from nightly "I think I'm going to die" panic attacks. It was a wholly unexpected, powerful, and much needed catharsis.

As I kept doing yoga, my heart opened, bit by bit. African dance opened my heart even more, deeply grounding me, as I felt the power of the drums and my feet on the earth. I learned to play guitar, and songs of pain and joy flowed through me.

Feeling purged and grounded, I was primed for what was next.

I felt drawn to take a Therapeutic Touch class, in which I placed my hands hovering just above my classmate with the intention to heal. Eyes closed, my inner vision was flooded with violet light. She felt it too. I was amazed and intrigued. My analytical mind wanted to understand it, while the budding Healer in me just accepted it with a knowing smile.

I joined a women's circle, and dove deep into the divine feminine: the earthy goddess energy felt like coming home. I had researched Reiki and was intrigued. So, when one of the women invited me to a weekly Reiki circle, I was excited to join. Receiving Reiki was fascinating. I felt waves of heat, or cold, and even an electric prickling. I could feel energy flowing: invisible, yet potent.

The next natural step, despite my painful hands, scientific questioning, and general skepticism, was to get my level one Reiki attunement. My inner skeptic wanted to brush it off as "woo-woo". But I couldn't ignore the fact that my experiences kept illuminating that there was more to life, and perhaps our spirits, than what I could see. Plus, by this time my eczema had expanded beyond just my hands, to the backs of my knees, my hips, and my breasts, all of it excruciatingly itchy.

So I stepped onto the Reiki path wholeheartedly, open-minded and ready. I resonated with the Reiki Principles, which instruct one to live in the present moment, with compassion, while offering one's talents to the world. The attunement itself felt odd, as I sat there, eyes closed, aware of the teacher mumbling, tracing secret symbols into my hands, and blowing air behind my head. My skeptical, agnostic mind sat in the corner and laughed.

And yet, I felt changed. My hands felt hot, though they were normally cold. I felt energy flowing through me, as if a faucet had turned on. I nudged my skeptical mind and my ego out of the way, placed my hands on a classmate to practice, and let the Reiki energy flow where it was needed. I felt it. The receiver felt it. And, most convincing of all, my eczema began to heal.

At first I thought it was the usual ebb, a brief reprieve from itching. I expected the itching to start again... anytime. But it didn't. The swelling subsided. The patches on my body went away entirely. Within 2 days, my hands looked and felt normal, though warmer and buzzing with energy. My analytical mind could not deny that my hands and body healed much faster than they "should" have. I have never had eczema on my body since, and my hands have never returned to their previous state.

Miracles were not part of the narrative of my upbringing. But what else could I call what I had experienced? "There must be a scientific explanation!" cried my inner skeptic, no longer laughing in the corner.

Perhaps, holding on to victimhood for so long damaged my hands. Maybe the burning and itching was my fear, pain and dis-ease, and all that remained was to let go. Literally, to open up my hands, allow healing to flow through me, from earth and sky and universal energy, gather it in my heart, and allow it to channel out through my hands.

I let the energy flow, and felt the irritation that had plagued me for years wash away. I felt a subtle, yet profound shift, like I had been a damaged piece of plumbing full of sludge, and was now a conduit, clean and new, with energy flowing and the ability to send it to others for their highest good.

It's believed that Reiki raises the frequency of the individual receiving an attunement. Perhaps, in raising my frequency, I became incandescent - my flame began, finally, to burn hot enough to incinerate the irritation of abuse and trauma, allowing me to become fully myself and paving the way for me to become the Healer I was born to be.

My newly healed hands made it possible to fully embrace my interest in massage. I became a Licensed Massage Therapist and have practiced massage and energy healing for the last 22 years.

Visiting my parents at a time when I was practicing my new Reiki skills, and feeling highly sensitized, I noticed that their relationship energy felt unbearably stagnant, and I spoke up. I told them I wouldn't visit again until they got counseling. My mom filed for divorce within the month. After 37 years of marriage, she was finished with being passive and allowing my dad to dominate her.

When she began speaking up for herself, my mom blossomed. For the first time in my life, I was finally able to get to know her. She surprised me often with new things she was excited to try: tai chi, dance, and even a ride in a hot air balloon. She exuded joy. I'm grateful to have had the last 12 years of her life to learn who she really was, once she was free to be herself.

My dad survived the divorce, despite suicidal moments. He grew in his own way, as he traveled in his RV. Though he spent the rest of his life hoping my mom would take him back, they remained friends. Both stayed single for the rest of their lives.

While I was in Massage School and my parents were in the midst of their divorce, I also studied second degree Reiki. The timing was perfect. I learned to send Reiki over space and time, to my parents, and even to myself as a child. Holding a picture of your self as a child and sending unconditional love and healing energy is one of the precious Reiki gifts I love helping others experience.

I was content with my Reiki training, and didn't think I would go on to become a Reiki Master. That calling came later, after the loss of my mom.

She was weeding around the blueberry bushes on the day she collapsed when a brain aneurysm burst: the last email we received from her was about the pill bugs she saw on the ground under those bushes, rolled up and looking like blueberries, and her amusement at how blue they were. She must have sent the email, and then collapsed as she walked back to the garden, dirt still under her hardworking nails.

I can still picture her hands, one week later, folded on her chest, holding a pink rose, placed there by the hospice nurses. As I sat with her body, I was surprised to feel her presence for the first time since that email. The intervening week of ICU, life support, and impossible decisions drifted away as I sat in the midnight hours with my mother's body, yet felt her spirit there with me at last. I talked to her then, and felt a sense that she would be nearby, even though she was physically gone.

While her death was as gut wrenching as it was unexpected, it was also a rite of passage that I was unaware existed until I was in the midst of it. It was as if I finally was cut loose from the body that grew, nurtured, and birthed me. At 41 years old, steeped in grief, I felt untethered, and surprisingly free to grow even more fully into my role as a Healer. The divine feminine voice that had gestated within me for years was clear: it was time for the next level of Reiki training. I was ready.

Now, when I place my hands on my clients, I feel my mom's presence as one of my helpers. I felt her while receiving my Reiki Master training. At a weeklong retreat, I felt her presence: sensing that she was giddy with excitement about the deep energy healing I was there to learn. I couldn't help but smile. I feel her by my side when I teach and attune my own Reiki students.

My teenage self wouldn't even recognize my present self. I have become one of those openhearted people I was so mystified by. When I say "Namaste", I truly mean it: the light in me sees the light in you. Over time, I realized I had a choice: remain skeptical and judgmental, or simply believe in the wonder of life. The fact is, I was changed, I accepted that change, and I chose to find meaning in my experience. In doing so, I became a Healer.

My hands that were once so abhorrent to strangers had become healing channels when I placed them with intention for the highest good, unconditional love, and the belief that miracles are possible. Although I would love to understand the "why" of Reiki and energy healing, I have learned to be at peace with simply accepting the mystery.

Reiki transformed me, showed me miracles are possible, and illuminated my calling as a Healer. Transmuting the painful experiences of my life into soulful gifts fueled my own metamorphosis. After all, a butterfly cannot emerge without first dissolving and reforming anew.

So what do I hope you, dear reader, come away from my story with?

I hope you see a glimpse of yourself in me, and through that mirror, find inspiration.

Perhaps you are reminded of the skeptical or miraculous moments in your own life.

Maybe you can look at your hands with renewed wonder.

You may be inspired to go outside and wiggle your toes in the grass, to breathe deeply and feel the earth beneath your feet.

Or maybe you are ready to cup that fading photo of yourself as an innocent child lovingly in your hands, and send that love back through the years.

I especially hope you can see that we all have the ability to learn and grow more fully into ourselves, no matter our set of beliefs.

If a skeptic like myself can experience miracles, anyone can. The miraculous is around us at all times - in our bodies, our communities, and our world. All it takes to sense miracles is a shift in perspective: one step, out of your own way, with open heart and hands, into infinite possibility.

About Hyla L Hitchcox, LMT

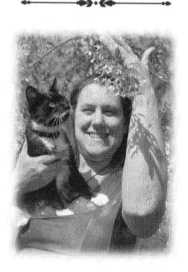

Hyla L Hitchcox, LMT, Reiki Master, has a BA in Humanities and BS in Environmental Studies. She lives in Pickerington, Ohio with her husband, two children, cats, chickens, fish and a turtle. She previously taught environmental education on board a tall ship and in the lush forests of her native Pacific Northwest. Her deep love of nature and the arts infuses her calling as a gifted, intuitive Healer. A Licensed Massage Therapist since 1999, Hyla also teaches qigong, yoga, and Chakradance.

She loves gardening, Taekwondo, and playing Zimbabwean style mbira and marimba music. Hyla offers virtual intuitive healing sessions, including deep grounding, meditation, movement and Reiki to heal the child within.

Follow her on Facebook: Hyla L Hitchcox, LMT, Reiki Master at: https://www.facebook.com/hyla.hitchcox

Chapter 14
Learning to Belong to Myself

Martha Chabinsky

In the past, his wide-eyed leer and awkward remarks caused me to keep my distance from him. Physically, I never touched my father-in-law except out of familial obligation. I attended holiday celebrations and Sunday dinners where I could taste his arrogance along with the food on my plate, and I just barely managed to keep from verbally reacting to Irv's egotistical diatribes.

Sixteen years later, I found myself caring for all his physical needs as he lay bed-ridden in the apartment we had created in our garage for *my* father. Irv was incontinent, and on a feeding tube and oxygen, so I had a lot of work to do just keeping those systems running well and him clean. I arranged and administered his medications, kept appointments with his doctors, and worked with the home health nurses who came to check on him. Deeply rooted in the present moment, the daily chores and trial-and-error of caring for a seriously ill person took over my life. Despite the awkwardness between us, him having to abandon his independence and privacy, and me being unable to forget his cruel words and disregard for the feelings of those around him, together we created a liturgy of his daily care.

The feelings of discomfort as I did what I considered to be my duty and cared for my father-in-law were, I thought, a relatively small price to pay for the possibility that my husband could experience a kind of closure to this difficult relationship he had with his Dad.

One day Irv asks us to take him to the Emergency Room. He is exhausted from all his ailments and waiting for the hospital staff to determine the next steps in his care. Standing next to his gurney, bored from the usual interminable ER wait, I look down and notice his hand resting on the white sheet that covers his body. It is dry, discolored from IVs, and worn from all the years of both duty and pleasure. I can sense his disconnection from all the activity going on around him, and feel compelled to connect, thinking maybe a little consolation might ease this moment for him. So, I lean over and whisper "Is it okay for me to rest my hand on yours?". Eyes still closed, he gives a tiny nod of approval and I gently lower my left hand onto his age-spotted right one.

This moment was not particularly meaningful to me at the time, just a blip on the six-week screen of the time he lived with us, and I never heard from Irv one way or the other about it. As it turns out, it was a singular moment of clarity which I later recognized as one of an empath, responding to a Divine nudge from deep inside myself.

My days were filled with family visits, drug store runs, keeping track of Irv's medication schedule, my own family's meal preparations and my youngest child's need for help with the structure of his life. At 15 he didn't want much to do with his grandfather, having been wounded by callous remarks about who Irv loved and didn't love, and so he kept his distance from all the activity surrounding Irv and his needs.

I sometimes felt overwhelmed with too many responsibilities, yet, at the same time, I noticed that the daily rituals of caring for another also have their comforting side. I found rhythm in the quiet, the gentle methodical actions, the time to observe and reflect while waiting for the nurse to arrive or the tea kettle to whistle, hearing birdsong outside the window by the bed, or a bit of music from the radio in the next room. These small gifts are generally lost in the worry, angst, and busyness of life, but occasionally they created a small oasis of calm for me, and perhaps for Irv too.

Using a baby monitor to communicate with Irv when he needed a diaper change or help getting into a different position in bed, we were awakened many times during the night. With a flashlight illuminating the pertinent parts, we had several moments of hilarity while cleaning him up, wondering what we would have thought if we had known years ago that this situation was in our futures. Laughter and smiles in the night can also bring calm and peace.

After Irv had been with us for six weeks, he was admitted to the hospital again, and I joined my husband on a visit to see his Dad the first night of his stay. It was unusual for me to do so because I needed a break from the constant care Irv required, but we had planned to shop for a new sofa afterwards, so I tagged along. When we walked into his hospital room, the nurse was having a tough time getting an accurate blood pressure reading as it was quite faint. She remarked that it had been this way for an hour or so.

Irv lay in his bed, cheeks pale and sunken, mouth agape, with one eye slightly open, the eyeball rolled up. His breaths were so far apart, it was impossible to know which was the last one, until there were no more. I touched his shoulder. We called to him, and then, he was gone. I had seen people close to death before, but I had not been present at the actual moment of passing. To me it felt otherworldly and ethereal, but more remarkable was the fact that Irv had died not 5 minutes after I walked into his room. I knew; Irv had been waiting for me.

Our son happened to also be in the hospital at this time, fulfilling his responsibilities as a volunteer. We called him up to Irv's room, and the three of us spent a half hour sitting together in that point of silence at the middle of the spiral we had been traveling with Irv. We returned home together and spent the evening in quiet pursuits, each of us going to bed early.

"Women are the vessels of the Mother Goddess," Jean Shinoda Bolen says in *Crossing to Avalon*. "Through reverent touch that is both personal and transpersonal, they accompany those who are passing into and out of this physical world." When I read this later in my life, I immediately remembered this first death experience and how it did not feel scary but felt deeply significant to me.

The typical sorts of tasks filled the next few weeks: removal of the rented hospital bed, disposal of Irv's many medicines, arranging for the cremation, and the transportation of his ashes to my husband's brother. This time was not without intensity and confusion either. We had quarrels with family members over financial dealings, and disagreements with doctors from Irv's previous location in Florida about bill payments and Medicare charges. It was a mess, but as all things do, it eventually passed and our lives returned to relative normalcy.

While eating lunch a few months later, I was leafing through the Main Line School Night catalog, and a course listing caught my attention: Therapeutic Touch. The description said: Learn how energy passing through our hands has the potential to calm and heal others. My last schooling experience had been high school, and I was never a keen student. I had never taken a night school course just for fun, but this course was about hands, and I remembered my intense desire to rest my hand on Irv's parched, quiet, old one. I signed up that afternoon.

Excited about learning something new, in class I discovered that the palms of our hands contain energy centers that when rubbed quickly together generate a magnetic feeling between them. Watching my class-mates practice on each other I was mesmerized by how hands tell more about a person than their face ever will: the gestures they use, how they convey love and caring, how capable working hands look beautifully powerful, and how in ballet or art hands have a graceful, light quality about them. Through watching hands in class, I fell even more deeply in love with them as they went about their work of experiencing the energy passing through their partner's body.

Learning this embodied practice as well as alternative healing modalities and Shamanic Journeying in two other classes I attended, I found myself gradually shifting from a completely allopathic understanding of medicine and health to a new understanding of vibration, intuition and a transpersonal, that is, a more spiritual, state of mind.

In the years leading up to this experience with Irv I had been expanding my reading to include more spiritual and natural-world concepts. Amongst others, I read Riane Eisler's The Chalice & the Blade and Jack Kornfield's A Path With Heart.

I filled journals with tarot and animal card readings, I learned everything I could about astrology, wholistic health practices, gardening, and in my daily journal I noted my desire to write about my experiences. I was waking up to something deeply embedded within me. I was listening to the voice inside, the one that told me what was right for me, and how to live life according to my own needs rather than the needs of others.

Practicing Transcendental Meditation for 20 years and reading Yoga Journal regularly, inspired me to start a yoga practice, and so the next class I signed up for was Kripalu Yoga. It was held in a high school gym and taught by a man by the name of Hari. In our first class, he demonstrated "meditation in motion," a practice in which a yogi/yogini allows their body to move into and out of postures without conscious intention. I'd never seen anything like it, and I was mesmerized by his introverted reflexive flow of ecstasy; this is, what it feels like to stand inside of one's self.

Something about it reminded me of the experience in the hospital, of answering an inner call, and I longed to have that experience again. It felt like a homecoming. In that first class I practiced Therapeutic Touch on myself and gained relief from a long-standing ache along my spine. I left class that evening high on love, for my new experiences, for taking care of myself, and for the growing and learning I was doing.

I attended every class in the session, and after it was over, Hari extended the class by teaching in a student's apartment. By this time, it was summer and quite hot in Pennsylvania. This student's apartment was on the 5th floor, and we practiced on a beautiful Oriental wool rug in her living room. Oddly, there was no air conditioning, and soon after we began, I was sweating profusely and feeling weak.

I told myself to keep doing the poses, but then I began feeling light-headed. When I thought I might faint, I finally complained about the heat. Hari scowled and admonished me to "let go of your desires and judgment and continue with the practice anyway." I simply could not relate to what seemed a narrow, confining, mind-over-matter approach. I wanted to listen to my body, to be directed by what I felt, not be told by an outside 'authority' what to do. Surprising myself, I rolled up my mat and walked out of that class!

Later, in mulling over everything that happened that evening, journaling about it and talking to a few special friends, it dawned on me that letting go of thinking I should do what Hari said was a dissolution, a death, and listening to the voice inside myself was a birth. This was the beginning of the transition into my understanding of the Divine Feminine as the inner guide of my life.

The next few years were a watershed time for me. As a member of my Unitarian-Universalist church I taught a Divine Feminine-based course called Rise Up and Call Her Name, in which I recognized that I was a Medicine Woman, a woman with a natural connection to the Earth and other women, able to see the spiral path of clarity and resonance.

I directed the annual Women's Spirituality Retreat, taught Sacred Labyrinth workshops, and helped arrange for Margot Adler, author of *Drawing Down the Moon* to lead a workshop for the women of my church community. Most significant though, was the advice I received from both our family therapist, Fran, and my night school teacher, Victoria: "Martha," they said, not two weeks apart, "you need to reclaim your power!" At the time, I wasn't completely sure what this looked like, and it was a while before I remembered and followed their sage advice.

A few years later, in 1997, when my announcement that I would be moving to NH was met with dismay, I answered my friends' questions with my assurance that 'something is waiting for me there.' I even had a vision about teaching yoga in front of a set of French doors in our new house. I did feel that I was leaving a magically supportive group of women at my church, but I had connected to an ancient-feeling, insistent draw of knowledge inside myself, and I didn't question it.

After moving, I found a yoga class that fit into my schedule and attended for a year, loving every minute of my new yoga life. When my teacher injured her back, she asked if anyone could demonstrate postures for her. My classmates suggested me, much to my surprise, but I was secretly pleased and agreed to attending her 5 classes a week as her assistant. Standing at the front of the class alongside my teacher I felt perfectly aligned with my soul. I was teaching yoga!

I had heard about Kripalu Center, just a couple of hours from my home, where my teacher had done her training. In reading the YTT (Yoga Teacher Training) course description I realized that Kripalu was perfect for me. The heart-based soft power of the compassionate approach to teaching that it described felt welcoming to me. This was a wildly new path, but it felt destined and perfect.

Everything that happened to put me on this path since I had laid my palm on Irv's hand in the Emergency Room of Bryn Mawr Hospital occurred without my direction or intention. It was easy and perfect, providential even. My Kripalu open heart began its journey that day with Irv, of all people. I just followed it.

Since completing teacher training more than 20 years ago, I have dedicated my practice and my teaching to the Divine Feminine in all of my students, male or female. Specializing in pre- and post-natal yoga for 10 years, teaching Goddess Yoga workshops and creating opportunities for my students to listen to their bodies and heal their spirits from the challenges of ordinary life, I feel I have been fulfilling Her instructions of honoring our bodies, learning from them and respecting their wisdom. Irv began to teach me this the day he accepted my touch.

It is what my teachers showed me as I gained knowledge through courses and trainings. It is what my students teach me as they trust me to be present for their own unfolding. Being a yoga teacher is a collaborative experience, just as it is to keep the Divine Feminine as my greatest guide.

Accompanying Irv as he walked toward his death, and students as they let go of old roles and habits to lean into new paths and ways of being, I am awed by the perfection of the world and all the experiences I have had here.

About Martha Chabinsky

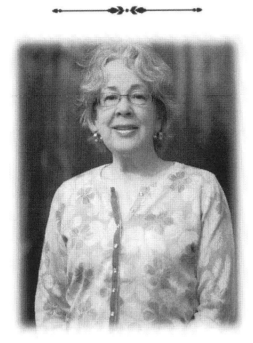

Martha Chabinsky has been teaching Kripalu yoga, with a specialty in pre- and post-natal yoga for over 20 years. She incorporates Reiki and Therapeutic Touch into her teaching repertoire whether it's in a workshop setting, her online offerings, or her weekly email. Her intention is to support and nurture the feminine in all students by creating opportunities for them to live inside their embodied truth.

As a master gardener and expert knitter, she brings a sense of creativity and fun to her teaching and sharing within her community. At work on her memoir of growing into understanding the presence of the Divine Feminine within herself, she spends each day relishing the natural world and all its gifts.

Blog: http://renaissancemoon.wordpress.com Join her email list and receive a free gift of December EnLIGHTenment, a holiday email celebration, at mchabinsky@gmail.com

Chapter 15
Daughter of Devotion

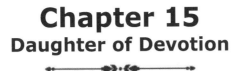

Jennifer DeVille Catalano

When I was in third grade, the school principal told my mother I had "the calling." Given that I attended parochial school where the principal was a nun, the vocation to which she was referring was the sisterhood. Though not an especially pious child, I did love the beautiful statue of Our Lady of Fatima in the back of the classroom as well as the rituals of Catholic Mass every Friday morning. Neither my mother nor I took Sister's comment to heart, though. We both knew I wanted to be a doctor and have a family someday. Becoming a Bride of Christ was not part of my life plan.

I received the sacrament of Confirmation and even became a Eucharistic Minister in high school, giving out Holy Communion at Mass. Nonetheless, I knew there was more to spirituality than I was being taught. I wanted to know about chakras, crystals, and hearing angels, but was terrified of being called a witch because Catholicism had labeled the New Age evil. A metaphysical bookstore opened within walking distance of my home and I delighted in all of the information to which I had access there. The owner told me she was named after Jeanne d'Arc (Joan of Arc), the French saint who had been burned at the stake for heresy, and that her intention was to provide a haven for people like her. It felt like a safe space for me, too.

Though I considered Religion as an undergraduate major, my love of foreign languages and travel led me on linguistic and literary paths to a Master's and then a PhD. On Labor Day 1999, I planned to enjoy a day of rest from my busy second year of doctoral study, but loud knocking awoke me just past six o'clock in the morning. I stumbled out of bed to find two policemen at my apartment door. What had I done?

My cheeks burned as they crossed the threshold. I respectfully declined their invitation to sit down, but ultimately acquiesced and balanced on the edge on my floral fold-out couch.

"Do you know someone named Ann?" one officer asked.

My vision went black. It was as though someone had thrown an opaque sheet over my head.

"That's my mom," I said into the darkness. In that same moment, I knew. "She's gone, isn't she?" I whispered.

"We're so sorry, ma'am," the other officer said. To this day I have no memory of what he or his partner looked like. I still couldn't see, but I could hear in a muffled, distant way, like someone was talking to me from the end of a long tunnel. The words "blunt impact" lingered somewhere between them and my consciousness.

"Did she suffer?" I couldn't bear the thought of her last moments being painful.

"No ma'am, she died instantly."

I sank into the void. There were no tears. There were no feelings at all, just obscurity. Perhaps seconds passed, or maybe minutes.

"How did you find me?" I asked. My mom lived in Ohio but was on vacation in California and there we were in my North Carolina apartment.

"She carried your name and number in her wallet."

Why me? At twenty-six, I was the youngest of her three children. I was honored yet horrified to inherit the job of informing my older siblings as well as my father, her ex-husband, of her death. I lived the news over and over and over again as I told them about Mom's fatal car accident.

Yelling, crying, questioning, and gasping for air filled my ears as each of them grappled with the greatest shock they had ever experienced. I just kept repeating the words the police officers had said to me, still not believing the news myself.

Each morning for close to a year, I awoke in a brief state of amnesia. After a few seconds, my world would go dim as my heart dropped all over again upon remembering my mother's death. The phone on my nightstand, the one I so often picked up to call her when I was scared and stressed-out, became another sign of her absence. For months I couldn't get out of bed before letting half of a tiny white anti-anxiety pill dissolve under my tongue. I sought regular counseling to keep my head above water as I continued teaching undergraduates, supervising teaching fellows, and attending graduate classes of my own. The magic of life was gone, though. I was barely managing to exist in a fog of suffering.

I explored many paths on my quest for healing, from pharmaceutical to non-traditional therapies. Eventually I found flower essences and a few vestiges of my younger self rose to the surface. Flowers were a bond I had always shared with my mom, from ordering daffodil bulbs by mail to picking out annuals at the local nursery together. In late spring each year, we filled the back of her car with flats of alyssum, geraniums, snapdragons, pansies and marigolds. Every May, my dad would help my siblings and me buy her a rose bush for Mother's Day. At the time, I didn't understand her love of roses. When I began working with flower essences, it became clear that rose is a flower of the heart. It is a flower of mothers that brings loving nourishment, soothes hurts, and encourages forgiveness. Rose is also the flower most often associated with Mother Mary, though after losing my mom, I felt little connection to my faith. I simply wanted relief from my heartache. Daffodil and rose were among the first flower essences I took, desperate for anything that could connect me to my mom and alleviate my misery.

The farther I got on my academic path, the more I shut down emotionally. My dissertation topic was about the lifesaving power of a woman's voice, yet I wasn't using mine authentically. I was spouting off literary jargon and presenting conference papers on obscure topics that had no impact on the real world. Finally, I reached my limit. Much to the chagrin of my advisor, I turned my back on the pursuit of a tenure-track job and moved to a Greek island, only flying back to North Carolina long enough to successfully defend the dissertation for which I wanted nothing more than closure.

Visiting ancient temples and working two summers at an archaeological dig on the island of Crete filled parts of me that were hungering for a bond with my mother and Mother Earth. At the same time, Orthodox Christianity permeated everyday life, revealing facets of Mother Mary I had never before seen. While I felt a reconnection to Mary in Greece, I had always been drawn to the goddesses of Ancient Greece and Egypt as well. My Catholic upbringing with the Holy Trinity of God the Father, Son, and Holy Spirit wasn't all-encompassing of my spirituality. During my years overseas, I began reading about Goddess religions. Yale-educated theologian Carol P. Christ, who relocated to Greece herself, was the first author whose work I read on the subject. I felt a definitive pull to return to the Earth and to a less dogmatic spirituality, but wasn't ready to be called a pagan. I continued to take various flower essences, yet kept them hidden along with the angel oracle cards I had bought at Jeanne's bookstore after my mom died. I knew the man with whom I was involved would call me a witch if he ever found them. Thankfully I finally left him, and moved back to the United States after succumbing to a severe case of mononucleosis.

Returning to my home country was deeply healing and grounding. The reinstatement of a more natural cycle of four seasons after almost five years in the Aegean climate consoled my being on multiple levels. During that time, I was also corresponding with a pen pal whose love of art and nature echoed my own. Months later, we met in person at a botanical garden in New York, and I knew he was the one. I felt an instant, deeper, more complete love with him than I had ever experienced. He was no stranger to grief, having lost his older brother in an accident many years prior, which helped me gradually and organically unearth feelings about my mom's death that I hadn't been willing to embody previously.

Having left academe behind, I settled into a storybook carriage house on Lake Ontario and started writing fiction. Walks along the water, bicycle rides with my beloved, and myriad creative pursuits filled my days. Then I found out, against all odds, that I was pregnant. Terror rushed through my veins. The Catholic girl in me felt ashamed because I wasn't married. The maternal orphan in me didn't want to give birth. How could I possibly mother a child when I hadn't healed from my own loss? At the same time, I had always yearned for a family, and I was deeply in love.

In 2011, Violet came into our lives with a strong will and a voice to match. She nursed around the clock and rarely slept more than twenty minutes at a time. The three of us moved out to the country, but her father continued to commute to the city for his night shift. My lack of sleep, utter overwhelm, and unprocessed grief took a serious toll on my physical and emotional wellbeing. I descended deep into postpartum depression, though I didn't know it at the time. I wasn't sad; I was angry and extremely irritable. I hated how hard life felt and I despised the fact that my mom wasn't there to help me navigate the turbulent territory of first-time motherhood.

Violet was eighteen months old when I emerged from the abyss in which I had been drowning and found my light again. Her father and I got married in our meadow of wildflowers and danced to Eva Cassidy singing "Fields of Gold." I wish my mom could have been there, and in a way, she was. Like an answered prayer, the clouds parted to reveal an enormous double rainbow after my husband and I had exchanged our vows. When my son was born thirteen months later, I no longer felt broken by motherhood. Violet had bravely paved the way for Oliver, the little Libra who brought balance and completion to our family.

One September afternoon in 2014, I went outside with my children to bask in the gleaming sunlight. As Oliver was crawling in some fallen leaves, Violet gifted me a handful of white asters that she had picked from her garden, along with one bright orange zinnia. The comforting energy of the asters combined with the childlike playfulness of the zinnia and traveled straight through the portal of my heart. I instantaneously set the flowers down on the rock retaining wall and arranged them into a simple mandala, adding four golden locust leaves. It wasn't a fancy work of art; it was an offering of genuine gratitude. We were warm, healthy, safe, and together, surrounded by natural beauty. That spontaneous mandala expressed the deep connection I felt to my children, my husband, Mother Earth, and my mom.

Creating mandalas with flowers culled from my daily nature walks became a devotional practice for me. I hadn't attended Mass in years, but I felt aligned with Divinity when "praying with petals," as I called it. I had always loved the cycles of nature, and mandala-making enabled me to synchronize with the changes and messages of Mother Earth. I began sharing my creations on Instagram along with descriptions of the flowers I had used and their energetic properties, which eventually led to local gallery exhibitions and sales of my work.

Although I had grown up learning how to identify many plants from my mother, the number of wildflowers I still did not know astounded me. At my feet lay new buds and blossoms calling to be noticed, some so petite the eye could easily pass over them. One tiny flower in particular ignited memories in me that I had long forgotten. Even though the lawn surrounding my childhood home was kept green, weed-free, and manicured by a landscaping company, there were some small bluish flowers far in the backyard that crept over from the neighbor's property. Back then, I loved to sit in that patch, feeling held in a timeless embrace of wonder, magic, and utmost calm. Spotting a few of those same flowers hidden in the grasses of the meadow where I live now reunited me with parts of myself that had still been buried in the heavy soil of grief. I brought a sprig of it back to the house and immediately began leafing through my copy of the *National Audubon Society Field Guide to North American Wildflowers*. At last I found her: Veronica. This wasn't the spiky veronica I had seen in nurseries, though; this was a type commonly known as speedwell. The creative fairy-lover I was as a child wiped the sleep from her eyes and reminded me how fun it is to play with flowers. Nature had always felt healing to me, and in creating mandalas with flowers, I started to attune myself better to what they had to offer. As an essence, common speedwell calms chaos, which might explain why I had felt so soothed and supported lying in a patch of it as a child. It is also wonderful for the intuition as well as for inhabiting the present moment.

Flowers and their essences became an even bigger part of my life as time passed. I had been taking part in a monthly experimental flower essence program for years, and was repeatedly amazed and enchanted by their healing properties. I even followed an unexpected inner whisper to create and lead nature-based library programs for helping children get to know their feelings and shine their bright lights in the world. Between teaching, writing, and having a family, my life felt very full. Then I received sudden and surprising guidance from that same mysterious voice to begin playing crystal singing bowls and leading women's circles. It made no logical sense. I was completely unable to read music let alone play it. Even the nuns in grade school knew I couldn't carry a tune to save my life. I had only been chosen as a song leader at Friday Mass once. They never made that mistake again. But there I was, feeling undeniably and lovingly prodded by that mysterious Divine Voice to take another big leap of faith. It would mean relinquishing my controlling, thinking brain yet again and trusting my heart to lead the way.

I soon became a distributor for my favorite flower essence and oil company, and was invited to teach children's yoga at a brand new studio. I agreed and asked to start holding New Moon and Full Moon women's circles there as well. I purchased my first set of quartz crystal singing bowls and trusted my intuition that everything would fall into place. Indeed it did. All of the praying and meditating I had done over the years, combined with my studies of chakras and flower essences, came together serendipitously. I led four beautiful women's circles around central nature mandalas I had built, then the coronavirus pandemic of 2020 was declared. Suddenly my family and I had to sequester at home. When I discovered thyme-leaved speedwell, a different species, blooming in the yard, I received the sign to trust in Divine Timing.

Schools shut down and it took a couple weeks for virtual learning to get organized. While searching online for math and reading exercises to keep my children engaged, I somehow came across *The Way of the Rose: The Radical Path of the Divine Feminine Hidden in the Rosary* by Clark Strand and Perdita Finn. I still don't know what clicks landed me there, but I knew I had to have that book. I learned that Strand is a former Buddhist monk who receives monthly visions of Our Lady of Woodstock, urging people to pray the rosary. Reading *The Way of the Rose* synthesized everything I had ever thought, felt, wondered, and believed about Divinity. Flowers, feelings, and prayers wove together in my consciousness without the oppression of religious doctrine or the threat of being called a witch. I had finally found the Mother. She is Mary but she is also known by many other names. Through the rosary, which was originally a garland of roses, everything literally came full circle for me. I dug out the crystal rosary my mother's parents had given me for my First Communion in second grade and began to pray the Hail Mary on my daily nature walks. The flower mandalas I had been creating all along were tangible rings of prayer.

When schools reopened in September, my children went back to in-person learning and I resumed my women's circles at the yoga studio. I also began offering sacred sound baths with upgraded alchemical crystal singing bowls. I start each session with grounding to Mother Earth and praying, as well as connecting to the Universe/God/Source/All That Is. Sprinkled throughout my classes are always flowers, in their physical form as well as their essences and aromas. Long before I bonded with my own mother through flowers, people prayed to the Divine Feminine through flora in the form of offerings, gardens, and strings of blossoms. Flowers are a conduit for connecting with the Mother. She is Mother Earth, the Divine Mother, Mother Mary, my own mother, and the mother in me. We are all connected.

Prior to my opening prayer for a sound bath in March 2021, I showered my clients in floral mists and urged them to speak and tone with their own voices as part of the healing process. I jokingly mentioned how I had an unused PhD, but that my doctoral dissertation was about the lifesaving power of a woman's voice. At that very moment, the "Share Your Voice" card flew from the lightworker deck I had been shuffling. I audibly gasped and my hands began to shake from the sudden realization that earning my PhD wasn't all for naught. It gave me the courage to leave academe; to get out of my head and into my body, using my senses to the fullest. Everything I had experienced, from Catholic school to graduate school to losing my mother to becoming a mother myself, had brought me to where I am now in Divine Timing. Each step has been a petal in the flower mandala of my life thus far.

I am not a nun, yet Sister's assessment of my calling almost four decades ago wasn't wrong. Though I became a doctor, wife, and mother as my mom and I anticipated, I feel deeply called by Divinity through the flowers, feelings, and sacred sounds of Mother Earth. I say at least one hundred Hail Marys on my daily nature walks, not out of duty, but out of devotion. I am no longer afraid to be labeled a witch for my beliefs and actions. I use my voice to help others, especially women, feel safe enough to leave the abstraction of thought and lead embodied lives of prayerful practice. Each time I mist my clients with roses, the Divine Feminine arrives, and when I gaze upon a field of daffodils, I enter that liminal space of past, present, and future where the Divine Voice can be heard. Whenever I get frustrated with the fast and furious world in which we live, thyme-leaved speedwell's message of Divine Timing soothes me. And so I walk rather than run, following the petals along my path, always held by the Mother in her many forms.

About Jennifer DeVille Catalano, PhD

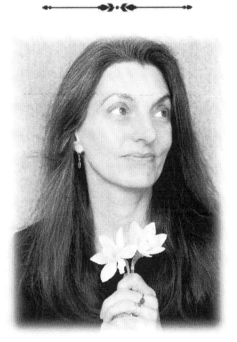

Jennifer DeVille Catalano, PhD, is a writer, artist, educator, and sound alchemist who believes everyday life is both luminous and numinous. Her deep love of nature permeates everything she does, from teaching children at local libraries to leading women on healing journeys both online and in person.

Jennifer marries sacred sounds, flower essences, and aromatherapy with contemplative practices and yoga to offer multi-sensory classes that facilitate healing. She lives in rural New York with her husband, two young children, two cats, and a multitude of wildflowers.

Visit her online at jenniferdeville.com, on Facebook at facebook.com/jenniferdevillecatalano, and connect with her via Instagram and Twitter as @jenniferdeville.

FULLY HUMAN — FULLY DIVINE

Chapter 16
My Life Path as a Divine Conduit

Lydie Ometto

My Journey

In Brazil, I grew up in a very loving family, the middle child of three children. My parents were deeply involved with spirituality. My dad was a channeler. He would receive information and write it down with his eyes closed (a form of channeling known as 'psychic psychography'). My mom was deeply connected to prayers and intuition. When I was between six and seven years old, I started receiving messages and seeing things that were not in the physical realm. I had the ability to see dead people. Please don't frown just yet. I can attest that this was something very natural for me, and "scary" was not a word I used to describe that time. As a matter of fact, it was quite comforting for me to connect with that world.

Once my parents recognized that I had started developing the ability to see non-materialistic things, they were supportive and urged me to connect to a group of adults who were studying and practicing spirituality. There were several channelers in this group, but the majority of the adults in it could not 'see' in the way I was seeing. Being a child, I was free of preconceived ideas, which helped me to be a clear channel. As I started going more frequently to the group, my capabilities started to increase.

I clearly remember many beautiful and powerful moments during the group meetings. One night, the spiritual readings were about love, compassion, and forgiveness. Red rose petals materialized over the table. Another time, one of the adult channelers let out a scream during the meditation prayer, and at that moment, as the whole group looked at her, pieces of broken glass materialized all over her face and on the table in front of her. We all kept on sharing 'psychic love', and in a matter of minutes, the glass disappeared. Later, we learned that at that exact time, a young woman had gone through her car's windshield 4 blocks away.

So for me, as a young girl, it was fascinating to be able to see people who had died recently or many years ago who were still stuck in limbo, so to speak. They were no longer in this physical realm, but they had not transitioned to a different sphere of life quite yet. Some were attached to family or to actions or consequences of their actions here in the living world. Some didn't believe that they had died.

Since I was so young, I didn't have the maturity or the knowledge to converse with them and explain their situation. These spirits would connect directly with me first, and then I would talk with the adults around me and say, "He's here, she's here, and they are saying this, this and that." Then the adults would help them to understand that they were no longer in their physical bodies and encourage and support them with moving on to the next chapter of their journeys. Some were grateful for the assistance and would go right away; some were a bit more difficult, and it could sometimes take more than a few days for them to move on.

For a period of six years, I did a lot of this work with the group. Also, in Brazil at that time, the group was very active in what they call spiritual surgeries—similar to the work of John of God (also Brazilian)—but in a smaller group.

Someone in our group would channel a doctor who existed in the spiritual realm, not the physical realm. These spiritual surgeons would support the embodied, living adults in our group. Many times, others would come to our group in extreme pain. I witnessed many of those surgeries because I was able to visually perceive the energetic aspects of the process.

I remember one woman came in with tremendous pain in her abdomen. One of the members of our group performed a spiritual surgery on her. It was almost like he used his finger as a scalpel. I could see blood energetically. Then it was like he reached his hand internally into her abdomen. I remember he pulled out something like a handful of hair, materializing the energetic-emotional stuff that she was holding in her abdomen. After prayers, and sometimes ceremony, the process was completed. There was no scar, and no more blood. Once that energetic material was removed, she was okay.

Personally, that time of my life also had a parallel side. At that age, I felt very different from my peers. I even remember arguing with my mom, saying, "I did not come from your belly. I was probably dropped off here by a spaceship or something else." She assured me and proved with pictures that I indeed came through her.

The energetic and emotional load was a bit much sometimes, so between seven and eight years old, I started going to a Yoga class with my very strong-willed French grandmother. Since I was dealing with so much on the spiritual realm, the classes helped me to ground and connect with the physical. That was also when I started connecting and experiencing the subtleties within the energetics of yoga.

Around age 13, my activity in the spiritual group was becoming too much for me. That part of my life was restricted to a small circle: my parents and the group. I was living two different lives. In one life, I was utilizing my gifts; in the other life, I was becoming a teenager. I felt alone and awkward. I was not relating well to my peers, and I couldn't explain it to them or their families. It was too hard for people to comprehend the expansiveness of my world, and hard for me to keep both aspects of my life running smoothly.

Around the same time, I started my menstrual cycle. Needless to say, I had so much happening physiologically and energetically that I decided to shut down the psychic part of my gift. For a couple of years, I did not play in that world anymore, except internally. I still had the capability, but I wasn't as open as I had been when I was younger.

Through this challenging transition, yoga was a support system for me, calming me down. Yoga allowed my mind to ground rather than be open to the messages from spirit.

Interestingly, although yoga can open you up to messages from spirit, at that time for me, it was the reverse. I experienced more stability and focus in the present moment. Again, it was beautiful that my parents and grandmother were there to support me, because if they had not been, I probably would have closed down my gift much earlier.

As a child, Yoga and my parents had supported me to open more, to assist and support others, and to handle my spiritual experiences inside of myself. Many times I saw things that were not suitable for my age. Some of the conversations were about why the people didn't want to disconnect from this world, and they were sometimes difficult topics to discuss.

For example, I channeled for a man who didn't want to leave because he said he had passed away too early. I don't remember if it was a car wreck or an illness, but he didn't want to accept that he had transitioned because he had young kids to care for, and two of his kids were very close to my age at that time. I also spoke for some who didn't understand that they had left this reality, because they had transitioned due to drugs, alcohol, or violence. It was interesting being there and listening, but some subjects were not quite understood by a child of my age.

When I first entered college, I majored in biology; I wanted to be a marine biologist. However, at that time in Brazil, marine biology was not popular. I realized that I would probably be stuck teaching in a tiny little room. I didn't want that, I wanted to be out there in nature, helping the ocean beings.

I shifted my major to physical therapy, and at the same time, started supporting people through healing touch and gentle hands-on work. I took extra trainings in everything that caught my attention: cranial sacral massage, Shiatsu massage, reflexology, and others. I even enrolled in acupuncture school. I was drawn to it, since everything that was supporting acupuncture had to do with energy. I thought, "This is fascinating! I can connect to the stars, the moon, the seasons and realize their effects in everybody." This interconnection is the basis of acupuncture, energy, and life.

This amazing phase of studies and growth assisted me in reconnecting with my gifts. I resonated with the energetics in all of it, soon adding Reiki and other modalities in which I utilized my psychic gift and my intuition through my hands.

At this time, I was also diving into the world of yoga in a deeper way, increasing my awareness of what was happening inside of me, and learning to deepen my trust in my choices in this lifetime. Not for several years did I allow myself to fully reopen to the non-physical realms.

All this sounds amazing, but as I was learning, growing and expanding my knowledge, my socio-emotional self was being depleted. I was the young woman at the parties responsible for 'caring' for the friends who needed a lift to get home after too much drinking and fun. I was feeling and connecting to all that was happening around me, and I felt responsible for doing something about it — to assist as needed.

When I moved to the United States in my late 20s, I started working as a Physical Therapist (PT) and continued my 'learning career.' I was like a sponge; I couldn't study enough. After many years of a full-time job, I left traditional PT work and started working for myself as a licensed massage therapist, doing hands-on massage and healing work. I incorporated everything that I had learned, plus brought a lot of my natural gifts of sensitivity and energetic connection to my work. I created my own potpourri of modalities. I assisted my clients to heal, strengthen their bodies, and deepen their connection to nature, and to life. Now, as I reflect on my spiritual work from ages 7 to 13, it was always a part of me to be a support for people wherever they were in life.

The transition from full-time PT to being self-employed was bigger than it sounds. Working in traditional PT meant I had regular 8am to 5pm work with benefits and security. One day I said, "No. I cannot do this anymore." Financially, my life was completely different. I no longer had any benefits, and I did not have guaranteed work. It was scary, especially the gap between a place of security and entering the unknown. Thankfully, I had friends who supported me tremendously by reminding me both of my strength within as well as the trust I held in my choices of this lifetime.

In addition, I constantly reached for my spiritual books and was reminded that transitions, though difficult, are stepping-stones on the path to the next level of evolution. With that perspective, I felt even stronger in stepping forward, trusting my choices, and trusting in the moment.

Slowly, I started building up my practice, doing more and more of what I loved, including organizing and participating in Humanitarian Missions for the underprivileged around the globe. I offered my assistance through hands-on healing, human connection, and translations.

After several years of in-depth involvement in teaching yoga, I was in a position to create a yoga school. That was when I started offering teacher trainings, teaching others to become yoga teachers. I produced five yoga DVDs, created and published a book on mudras or yogic hand positions, and continued with my studies, my evolution, which eventually led me to became a coach and mentor to others. And here I am!

One thing just flowed into the next. It seemed like everything was being orchestrated. I may have thought that I was in control, but in reality, it was the belief in my moment-to-moment choices that supported this divine orchestration.

At the time of my transition to self-employment, I started a beautiful relationship. My partner was also very connected to spirituality and the metaphysical aspects of life. His support helped me to remember my inner strength, my inner power, and that confirmation of the divine orchestration of life.

Certainly, I had many moments when I was overwhelmed, insecure, and fearful. But once again, the spiritual teachings and my trust in life and the people around me were what pulled me out of those feelings. Right about the time of menopause, I experienced a high level of stress and anxiety. Yoga and breathwork helped tremendously. I remembered that this was an opportunity to trust my being and relax into my natural goodness.

Now, in my new physiological expression — the wisdom time of menopause — I am reopening to my intuitive gifts in a wiser way and with a deepening in my energetic awareness. I feel I have done much in my life, and gathering it all, I see life from a new perspective. This new perspective supports my belief in humanity and all life on this planet, which then gives me the courage to bring forth my gift.

As human beings, I have come to understand that we all have incredible intuitive gifts. Some people have a deeper openness to those gifts from an early age and some choose to develop them throughout life, as their life experiences lead them to an expanded openness and awareness. And as I do it, I know we all can do it by tapping into the power of our everyday choices.

At my retreats on Yoga & swimming with dolphins in the wild ocean, I share much of this energetic connection of life and intuition. These sentient beings can surely teach and assist us to remember our intuitive powers.

The beauty is that nowadays, more of us understand that humans are "Divine Beings having a Human Experience." This belief is much more acceptable within many areas of society. For that reason, more people are opening to their own intuitive gifts and remembering their divine capabilities.

Some Favorite Healing Stories

Louise has transitioned now. When I started working with her, she was in her late 60s, and had troubling knee and hip problems. I started using traditional PT and later added energy work, visualization, and my own intuition.

She began engaging with energy work after she experienced the profound transformation of her state of being. Being a religious woman, she found she was now able to connect to her angels in a deeper and new way. She told me that she was able to see her angels and things she never had seen before in her dreams. They told her to cook for the poor. They told her to smile every day. They told her that her presence was supportive for the ones around her.

Not only did she stop having knee and hip pain, but she also lost about 20 pounds. She went from lying around, not doing much, to opening up her kitchen to serve the underprivileged population in the area, especially the homeless. Having spent some of her youth in New Orleans, her favorite food was gumbo, so she used to make huge pots of gumbo and serve it to the homeless. They would come to the front of her house, where she had set up tables to feed them in her driveway. It was beautiful and inspiring.

Another of my favorite stories is about a young teenager who I worked with using both yoga and hands-on bodywork. She carried a great deal of stress and emotional trauma from her childhood. She worked with me for about four or five years during her transition from teenager to a young adult in her early 20s.

When I began working with her, she could barely open her jaws; she was only able to nourish herself by eating liquid food through a straw. She had been to dentists and surgeons, searching everywhere to find help, but nothing was working. I started teaching her guided relaxation and restorative yoga, in combination with hands-on massage, craniosacral and energy work.

Slowly we started using more postures to allow the energy to move through her body, and breathwork to process the emotions from her childhood. She improved enough to be able to decrease many of the medications that she was taking. She started feeling more comfortable in her body, and as she learned how to manage her stress, her body tension started to diminish, and much of her trauma started to turn into positive opportunities for learning. Bit by bit, she remembered how to smile.

As she nourished herself with a new way of thinking and seeing the world, her jaws started to open. She began to believe that she could nourish herself with food — not just liquid food through a straw. Everything started to open up: not just her jaws, but also her face, her shoulders, and her whole body — not only physically, but mentally, emotionally and spiritually. Once her jaws released, she felt liberated. She went to school, got a profession, and transformed her eating disorders. She found a vitality, enthusiasm, and love for life that she never knew was possible.

My Legacy

I support people to remember their birthright of joyfulness, embracing happiness, and the ability to connect to self and others. I help them remember their innate ability to connect with plants, animals and all life, to receive and give gratitude, and to offer open hands and support to others. I assist them in finding a moment of peace, a space for compassion, a will to feel strong and vital, as they experience life moving through their bodies with ease.

My desire is that I can inspire people to remember that we all have a soul connection. We might dress differently, talk differently, express differently, but no matter what, we are the same. We are all "spiritual beings having a human experience." In light, we are all connected.

Each individual has their own spiritual journey, which can be expressed in a variety of unique ways. The main point is that once we connect deeper to the spiritual understanding of our "human journey," we become more grateful for the everyday gifts of life. In events that we may perceive as "bad or good," we always have a choice of how we incorporate them into our lives. As we gain a deeper level of understanding, we can choose to be burdened or we can choose to see the Divine miracles in everything.

At this moment in time, we are on this planet embracing the fabric of creation in which each one of us, as an individual and collective thread, is important, necessary, and divine.

About Lydie Ometto, E-500RYT, RPT

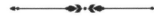

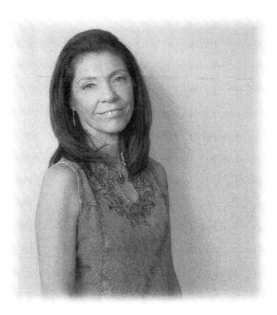

Lydie Ometto, E-500RYT, RPT, C-IAYT, sees Yoga as her passion. She is certified in Integrative Yoga Therapy, a Reiki Master and an Integrative Coach. Her background, as a Doctor of Physical Therapy, Massage Therapist, Acupuncturist (BR), Energyworker, and Breathworker, inspires her classes, trainings, sessions, and ceremonies. Lydie is the founder/director of InnerSeaYoga Teacher Training Programs. Her love of nature and overall Divine creation infuses her work.

As a wisdom keeper, she leads international yoga and transformational retreats, plus Yoga & Wellness Coaching programs. She is constantly deepening her studies in life, wellness, holistic living, women's transitions and joyful awakening, while reminding others to believe in their light.

Lydie's website is www.lydieometto.com. Lydie's gift to you: "The five essential steps to connect with your intuitive gifts"
https://www.lydieometto.com/intuitive-gifts-gift

Chapter 17
A Mayan Healer Finds Her Voice in a Foreign Land

Laura Hernandez

My earliest memories begin when I was only two years old. I was born in Mexico City. My roots there run deep, as my parents are descended from the Mayan people. This has always given me a strong sense of grounding. When I was five or six years old, I wanted to sing and dance, but something held me back.

For some reason, I was always very shy. I only had a few good friends. I loved animals and plants. I was always outside with the flowers, the dogs, and the cats. In Mexico, we live outside. That was our lifestyle.

I grew up striving to be the perfect student. I always had incredible grades and was considered the smartest one. I always completed my assignments. I was a perfect daughter. But I was also self-conscious.

The sense of something holding me back persisted. As I grew older, my shyness worsened, and that upset me. I would ask myself, "Why am I this way? I don't want to be this way. I know I'm more." But I hadn't yet found either the right people or the right place to express myself.

Life went on and I started broadening my studies. I took every kind of dance lesson. There was movement and some expansion in my life, and yet I was still the smartest one in class. I didn't want to be the perfect one in class because my friends were able to do what they wanted. They would say, "Oh, it's okay what I do because I'm not perfect. But you? Don't do this and don't do that because you're the smartest one." I got upset. I didn't want to be this person anymore. I didn't want to be the perfect good girl. I wanted to be free.

Time passed, and the shyness faded away. I started focusing my studies on a career. When I was 18 years old, I worked up the courage to tell my parents, "I want to learn English. I know we have some family in New York, and I want to go there." My parents' mouths dropped open, and their eyes widened. They were thinking, "What? This shy girl wants to go away to New York?" But, after a few minutes, they said, "Okay, we're going to support you in this."

Long story short, I went to New York to spend my summer with some relatives who I didn't even know. When I landed in New York, my aunt picked me up at the airport. She said, "Your uncle and I are getting divorced." I had just landed in the middle of a broken family, in the midst of getting separated, and fighting over everything. I had two choices— catch the next plane back home or stay.

In the deepest of loneliness that summer, crying, I asked myself, "Where am I? I miss my mom. I miss my dad. What have I done?" An answer came to me: "You're right where you need to be." So, two weeks of vacation in New York became a couple of months, and a couple months became a year. I took all kinds of dance classes. I got to know a cousin, who was a little younger than me. I became her big sister. I found my place, and I was really happy there.

I wanted to work in the United Nations as a translator, so I got in touch with people who worked there. They invited me to participate in some of the UN translation sessions. For me, it was a revelation: "Wow. This is what I want to do!" I went back to Mexico City and studied to be a translator and an interpreter. My whole career started because I was able to express what other people were saying.

I started working for the Canadian embassy. I was once again the good employee, one of the most highly qualified with all sorts of recognition. I became a trusted employee and I felt that I was really where I needed to be. I experienced many adventures during those years.

I was always very close to my grandmothers. They taught me how to access the natural way of medicine, and what it means to work with the earth, and spirits and angels—things that grandmothers tell you in stories. It made me uncomfortable, but I was curious.

In all of these years of work, I was very mentally focused in my profession and my career, but I was aware of little happenings and signs of something much more subtle. One of the first was when I went to a conference at the Biltmore Hotel in Florida. One night I was sleeping in my bed, and I suddenly woke up aware that there was somebody sitting next to me. I panicked and turned on the lights. Of course, there was nobody. Then I said to myself, "Okay, you're just dreaming. You're tired."

The next night, things happened that were not natural. The radio turned on. The lights came on. Frightened, I went to my friend's room. I said, "I have to sleep here tonight, in your room. My room is just too weird."

The next morning, we were told that the hotel was once a hospital and some energies were still there. I thought, "No, no, no, no...this is not me. I'm just dreaming. I didn't feel this. It's just too weird." This psychic awareness was the beginning of something that I had never considered I would be experiencing in my life.

Years later, I experienced more events. I was around 36 years old and living in Canada. Living in Mexico had gotten dangerous, and I just didn't want that for my family or future family, so I had left my Mexico, my dear country, and I went to Canada to continue my life.

One event, in particular, was very dramatic. I still get emotional when I talk about this. There was a little girl who died in an accident, a fire. When she died, I went to put flowers at the location of her death. My grandmothers taught me that when a child dies, you place white flowers, and so I did.

From that moment on, I felt this little girl was stuck with me. I would turn my head and would see her little head with her little dress. I would turn around and she was there. I wondered, "How do I make peace with this? What am I supposed to do?"

From somewhere...I heard voices, as if in a dream, telling me, "You have to help her because she doesn't know what to do." So, I talked to her and I told her that she could go. That was my first experience helping a soul find its way home. That's a big thing.

So there I was, a Mexican girl living in a small town outside of Montreal, Canada. I became co-owner of a fasting clinic with my partner where I worked during many years helping people through their process. I had endured many miscarriages, but then my beautiful, amazing miracle baby happened to choose me as a parent. Now I have a 15-year-old son.

I remember asking my mom, "What was my birth like?" She told me, "It was so cold that you would not have believed it was Mexico. It was snowing, which never happens in Mexico City." And then she told me "When you came out, the umbilical cord was around your throat. You almost didn't make it. You were all purple." The doctor said, "She's not breathing." But then, somehow, I came back to life and started breathing.

When my son was born, he too had the umbilical cord around his neck. I said, "No, this is not going to happen; not the same thing that happened to me!" They did everything to help me. When he came out, I took the umbilical cord and cut it, and said, "Okay, that's it." He was born healthy. Events like this make you wonder how they have shaped your life. Was this what I was always afraid to say, that I always felt I had something around my throat? Was this the something that was holding me back that I never was able to express?

I started putting things together. Sometimes I just want to say so much. I want to share what I know, and what I know is not what I learned at school. What I know are things that I learned from my grandmothers, and lessons from the forest, the animals, and beyond the physical realm of things. When I talk about this, it's confusing and it's deep. At the same time, it feels like it's truly me. It's not just a cover.

So here in Canada, I started working in international affairs and continued working in translation and interpretation. I was doing that and was really happy, but always looking for something more—another challenge in life.

When I took my first yoga class, I thought, "Oh, I like this." I liked all these shapes we put our bodies into and I felt like the energy became greater. I felt like I was coming out of an eggshell or emerging from a cocoon. Yoga helped me discover something more than just the physical body. For the first time, I connected with my expanded self. I felt something that I now call energy, beyond the borders of the physical body.

I continued to study with my Canadian yoga family. I dove into my studies and collected all kinds of certifications: therapeutic yoga, prenatal yoga, yoga after pregnancy, yoga for older people, and more.

Six years ago, when I started participating in Laura Cornell's Divine Feminine Yoga and women's circles, I told her my story. I recall a special moment when we were in a circle of four women. We were talking about our personalities and how we are in the world. Together, the women baptized me as 'Howling Coyote'. Resistant, I said, "That's not me at all.

That's the opposite of me. I'm not a howling coyote. I never speak up or howl—no way. A coyote is this free being in the forest." I thought, "Okay, I'll try to feel what it's like to be that coyote." I took the name with me, and began to try to understand its meaning for me.

Not long ago, my yoga career expanded. I left the international business side of my life, and I became a full-time yoga teacher. I now have the opportunity to speak out loud, as I guide my students through postures; but at the same time, I also say out loud what I feel and what I feel life is all about.

A new chapter of my life started once I became able to express what I know. I knew that I had to communicate it. Even now, when I speak my truth, I feel shivers down my spine. I know there's wisdom that I need to communicate to whomever wants to listen.

Yoga has brought me the opportunity to work with many different kinds of people. About five years ago, I started to make contact with people, some of them my students, who were suffering through cancer. I started studying and discovering the specific challenges of oncology yoga. As is my nature, I completed two certifications in this specialty. I can tell you right-side-up and upside-down what all the symptoms of cancer are, as well as medications that people take, and their side effects.

Several years ago, when I was teaching, I had a revelation: "I know why I had to do this. I'm not just teaching a body to put itself into yoga forms. I'm teaching yoga on a soul level. I'm talking to the soul that is in that body." For me, it became clear that I'm not just guiding somebody with a disease, but I'm also connecting to the person's soul or energy because they need guidance to go through something, to pass through something, or to evolve in some way.

It's now my passion, my mission, my pleasure, and my challenge. Sometimes I see people so very ill, and I know they're going to die. I sense it; I feel it. I know, when they don't come back to class, it's because they have passed away. I go through a lot of grieving, wondering why this person had to die. But then I just let go. I understand that when they were in front of me, even if their physical body had its challenges, maybe I said something that helped them, assisting them to evolve somehow, or transition to a new somewhere.

I respect life so much and I also respect death. In the teachings of the Mayan people, we celebrate death because it's just a transformation, another step on our path. Sometimes, when I talk about this, it's hard for people to hear. I'm very open with my thoughts to help others understand death in this way.

Some people have said, "Oh, you're the Mayan shaman." I don't want titles. I'm hesitant to call myself a shaman. I honor the word shaman from my ancestors because I know what a huge responsibility it is. I'm not looking for another certification from learning in school how to be a shaman. But, at the same time, I believe it's time for me to own that I am a healer, a Mayan healer in a foreign land.

I recently turned 53 years old. In my cultural traditions, when you are in or finishing your 52nd year, you celebrate having completed four 13-year cycles in your life. It means you have gone through many experiences in life: the child transitioning into the teenage years, in turn becoming a young woman, maybe a mother in the fertile times, and then caring for children. Now, becoming 53 years old, this is the time to express who we are. I'm going to celebrate with one of my women friends from my circle, Maria Magdalena. She was the midwife who delivered my baby when he was born. We will celebrate and perform a ceremony to celebrate my passing into this cycle, to completing all of my four cycles of 13 years.

In my culture and in many other cultures—not only the Mayan, but now also in Mexico—responsibility comes with this ceremony and celebration. As we move into a more mature state, we need to discover how and who we will serve. This is not about giving birth to a child or having a career or a profession or wealth or collecting fancy things. It's how you are going to serve in the remaining years of your life. This is what has been going through my mind. I'm preparing myself for this new phase of my life.

When I was a young girl, I used to sit on the balcony outside my house. There was a mountain far away, and I was always looking at that mountain. I was imagining myself being on that mountain, and wondering, "What is behind that mountain?" In that silence, I was able to see everything around me. All my traveling—all this moving from place to place over the years brought me to this little town just an hour from Montreal. Here, in the cold Canadian winters, away from my beautiful Mayan ocean in Mexico— sometimes I wonder, "What am I doing here?"

Then I realize that if I had never come here, I would never have found out what was behind that mountain. My travels started in New York, and then from New York to Montreal, and from Montreal to this small town. Now, my way of seeing is expanded; I see behind the mountain, and even farther away than just my own and others' physical bodies—with a wider perspective. In these difficult times that we are living through, we are all together. All one.

When I first came to Canada, I went through a very difficult breakup and separation with the father of my child. Since that time, much has healed. I now have a very nice, harmonious relationship with him and his family—a happy, content relationship.

I organize many women's circles here in my small village. Some call me 'the Mayan healer'. Some call me 'the shaman'. Some call me 'the little Mexican'. Some call me 'the witch'. Some call me just 'Laura'. I'm used to many names. One thing that I have to say is I always put my foot down in terms of finding my place here. I don't let anyone or anything step on my roots or who I am. It is very important for women—no matter where you are—to listen, to be aware of everything that is around you, but never, ever let anybody put you down.

I want to howl like a coyote: *Respect yourself and you will be respected*! We need to teach this to younger generations. I hope this message will serve my readers and they will say, "Okay, it doesn't matter how far from home I am. What is important is that I learn how to make my place wherever I am."

There's so much more to life than just being a physical body. But it's a responsibility and an honor to be a woman in this physical body. I reflect on what I've done in women's circles. We sing and dance. I have my yoga studio here in Quebec. I'm close to a lake. Sometimes I go into my little rituals on the lake: I bless the lake, lift water, talk to the lake and talk to the moon. Sometimes you may see me at midnight in the lake. That's when they call me a witch. But often, I can't avoid it. That's just me.

I'm happy. I've received a couple of recognitions from my community and from the city of Montreal. I never imagined it, but there is an organization from Montreal that works to encourage women in business. I received a social entrepreneur of the year award for my work with people who have cancer. In my community, I'm very humble. But people know what I do and they respect me.

For me, it is essential to be amongst other women searching for community. In the most trying moments, it sometimes is really hard to say, "Hey, I need help." In community, we find friends—sometimes people who we don't even know—who will just listen to us and support us.

For me, going through my divorce was a very challenging time. Having always been around other women, my grandmothers, women in my community, my teachers—I could tap into that strength.

My grandmothers are not alive anymore—but I have their pictures right here, and I feel the three of them smiling on me when I am searching for advice and support. You may not find what you seek in books, but always trust that you have resources where you can go and you will be heard.

You can pick up the phone, or you can sit down and meditate. Ask your guides, your angels, or ask your grandmothers—ask whoever you believe is there to help you. You will receive support. Sometimes we don't even notice it because it doesn't come in a message on your doorstep. It comes to you in other ways.

When you're really lost and you feel like, "I'm nobody. I'm a failure," let me tell you, "No, you are not." Just take a moment of silence. If you cannot be in silence by yourself, get somebody to sit down with you. You don't have to talk. Just sit down with another woman. Then, with feminine energy and trust in divine energy, things happen. Things open up. Don't be alone. I think if we don't find our voice and speak our truth, then we cannot fully be who we are.

About Laura Hernandez

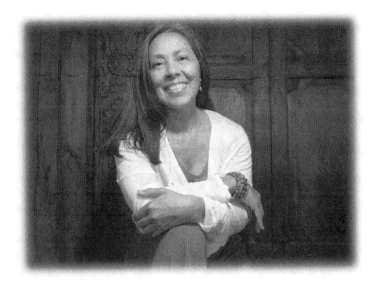

Laura Hernandez is the founder and owner of the Yoga & Movement studio. Prior to moving to Canada and founding Yoga & Movement, she worked as an international economic development officer from her native Mexico.

She has taught and practiced yoga for over 20 years. Her holistic approach allows students to increase strength and flexibility, both physically and mentally. Her natural patience, compassion, and calm energy provide a nurturing environment for this process. Her teaching and practice are influenced by the richness of her Mayan lineage.

Laura specializes in teaching oncology yoga to support people through cancer. Rituals of life and transformation are a part of her teachings.

"I don't talk to the body with disease but rather communicate with the soul and support her divine healing."

www.yogaetmouvement.com

Chapter 18
Sex and Love on the Path to Spiritual Growth

Laura J Cornell

I have longed for deep and authentic relationships my entire life, but as a young person, I didn't know how to have them. It took many decades of false starts for me to form bonds with others that would support my full spectrum growth and joy.

I grew up in a religion called Christian Science that did not honor the body, sexuality, or even normal human emotions. Christian Science insists on celibacy before marriage. I was given almost no sex education other than the basic facts of reproduction. Sexual pleasure was never mentioned and the words "gay, lesbian, or bisexual" were non-existent.

The trauma of being molested by my sexually-repressed father distanced me from my emotions and from connecting with others. I wrote about this trauma in my book, *Moon Salutations: Women's Journey Through Yoga to Healing, Power, and Peace* as well as in my book chapter, "#MeToo: How I Healed from Incest to Awaken to the Divine Feminine Within" in *The Game Changers* by Iman Aghay.

My three best friends in high school were all gay men. Two of them were secretly lovers, though I knew none of this back then. At the same time, I had a crush on my best female friend and was ashamed of my feelings, worrying that something was wrong with me.

Later, I would come to understand that I am bisexual. However, in high school, neither my friends nor I were able to give voice to our experiences or to be honest with ourselves, let alone each other. Despite our friendship, we remained isolated in our confusion. For me, at least, I know this was painful.

A part of me wanted to date, even though it seemed far out of my reach. In my high school senior year, I tried kissing a boy I liked, but I immediately froze in terror, as the experience reminded me of my dad. Without fully understanding what was going on inside of me, I called the boy the next day and said I didn't want to see him again.

First Steps in Opening the Energetic Constrictions

I met my first true love my sophomore year of college. He had a big smile and we connected instantly. We became lab partners in physics class and also good friends. One year later, coincidentally, we both took a non-credit, comprehensive course in human sexuality. This course changed the trajectory of my life, as I learned about the full range of pleasure, orgasm, contraceptives, gay and straight sex, intimate connection, communication, and boundaries.

By the end of the semester, Gary and I were deeply in love, exploring the bliss of all we had been taught in sex class. We were both virgins and I felt completely safe with him. Our time together was true joy, a form of play and celebration.

Through our slow, mutual exploration of pleasure, I released the constrictions I held around sexual sensation and expression. I allowed sensual energy to flow through my body and loved every moment of it. The incredible restriction inside me from childhood had a chance to heal. The blessing of that first sexual connection, so highly positive, flowed into all my later relationships.

Two years later the puppy love with Gary wore off. Something in me refused to settle, as I knew he didn't love the rabble-rouser, rebel side of me, the side that liked to dance and choreograph or to retake the sex class because it was so darn interesting. To be truly happy with Gary, I would have had to have become much more conventional than I was.

That wasn't even an option, so I told him I knew he wasn't my permanent love. We were both heartbroken over the loss of this blissful time together, but ultimately we parted ways.

The World is One Family

Two years after college, I moved to San Francisco and began to meet Latin American immigrants. My initiation into the injustices and indignities of cross-border realities was far from gentle, as I was with my first Latino boyfriend when he was deported.

We had gone to attend a hearing at the San Francisco City Courthouse for what my Guatemalan lover told me was a minor offense. Three heavily armed men approached us in the massive granite hallway, asking his name. They then handcuffed him and removed him abruptly through a side door.

One officer stayed in the hallway, looking at me. "Didn't you know?" he asked. "Know what?" I said. "That he's illegal." I stared at the officer in disbelief as the reality of what had just happened dawned on me. In my shock, in the loss of my companion, and in my concern for his well-being, I understood what it means to be "undocumented," and to live under the constant threat of being forcibly sent somewhere you truly don't want to be.

Though we were never a romantic couple again, something in me opened to learning more about his people and to doing my part to create a kinder and gentler immigrant experience. This relationship opened up a deeper part of my heart — that of caring about those who are very different than me.

I felt an immediate solidarity with those who are discriminated against, with people who come from poor countries, have browner skin, and vastly fewer economic or educational opportunities than I do.

Many years later, between my two marriages, I had a relationship with a Nigerian man. I feel strongly that the world is one family, and these experiences of dating across differences are part of what taught me that.

After the deportation experience, I began to learn Spanish, volunteered with refugee organizations, and spent multiple summers traveling to Mexico and Guatemala. I dated a Nicaraguan engineer and artist who had been drafted and fought in the Sandinista army, and who was still deeply traumatized by it. I fell in love with a man from Oaxaca, Mexico who was a high school English teacher by day and sang *Nueva Cancion* (New Song) by night.

People told me that I sounded like a different person when I spoke Spanish and I knew what they meant. This inherently romantic language brought out a more soulful, softer side of my personality than I had developed previously.

The men I dated honored this soulful side of me as well. One night during this time, I dreamed of a beautiful pot in my womb. I knew this was a vision of my femininity, my creative fertility being awakened. While I was connecting sexually with these men, I was also opening to my own feminine essence.

Dating Women

Just a few years later, I had my first female lover back in San Francisco. Yesica Maria picked me out at a party where I had played *Gracias a la Vida* (*Thanks to Life*) on the guitar and we became an item. She was drunk the first time we made love and I told her the next morning that I wasn't into that. "That's not a problem," she said. "I can stop drinking." Little did I know the ways of alcoholism.

It was a relief and a joy to finally be dating a woman because for a long time I had had crushes on women that didn't go anywhere. Making love with Yesica Maria felt like making love with honey. I loved taking her on adventures such as camping in the Sierras. I still remember her big smile shining out of the tent in the mornings.

Her alcoholism resurfaced after a few months though, and once I got over my shock and disbelief at her completely altered personality, I ended the relationship.

Soon after that I decided not to have a child in this lifetime, something I had always thought I wanted. I was increasingly aware of ecological and social crises faced by our earth, and I didn't think it was the best time to add another child to the planet. I grieved this decision, as I believed I would have enjoyed bearing a child.

At the same time, I was tired of falling in and out of love, which drained me emotionally. I prayed for a long-term partner, telling God/Goddess that whichever gender He/She brought me, I would be happy.

My next partnership would last 11 years. I call this my first marriage. Like me, Rose was spiritually oriented and into healthy living. I enjoyed our companionship, fun times, and mutual support. Rose was very social and we shared a wide circle of friends, which helped me to grow out of some of my social awkwardness.

The prayers I had put out for relationship stability had been answered, and the growth I experienced during those years was massive. My work in the world started to come into focus. I began to listen to my inner guidance and followed my bliss.

While I was with Rose, I became a yoga teacher, wrote my Masters Thesis on The Moon Salutation, did my dissertation research, and founded the Green Yoga Association. My blossoming yoga practice helped to open even more the free flow of energetic and sexual energy within me.

But there were challenges with Rose. I remember once after we had been fighting, I was praying at the Siddha Yoga Ashram. I sat with my head bowed in front of the statue of Baba Muktananda and I prayed inwardly, "Please help me. Look at how very reactive I am! What can I do about this?"

The response that came back was, "Teach the child to love." I took that as a reminder that it was my responsibility to guide my inner child in the direction of love, in the direction of maturity.

Over time I became clearer that Rose and I weren't happy together. I broached the subject with her, suggesting that we separate. She became very angry, and I wasn't clear or courageous enough to insist on separation in the face of her upset.

A few months later, I had a dream of a lingam, the Vedic symbol of a phallus. In my dream, the lingam took the form of a fountain. It stood upright, gushing water upwards. I felt awe at the innate creativity and energy of that form. I said to my companion in the dream, "I like that, I *really* like that." When I awoke I knew the meaning of this dream immediately. I, Laura Cornell, enjoy penises. I instinctively knew that should Rose and I separate, my next partner would be a man.

Three months after my phallic dream, Rose asked for my permission to have an affair. Thus began the unraveling that led to our separation. A heavy cloud of anger and resentment hung over me for months at the way our relationship had ended, but I eventually felt profound relief that it was over. I felt gratitude towards Rose for being the one to make it happen. We had grown apart, and it was time to move on.

Going for my Dreams

During that breakup year, I produced and co-directed the first Green Yoga Conference. I was also on deadline to complete and defend my dissertation. It was a lot, and I was busy.

At the same time, I longed to be dating. Every so often I would ask my inner guidance, *Can I start dating?* I very much wanted to hear a *Yes*. And every time, I would get the clear reply, *Not yet*. I sighed and surrendered. I waited.

About three months after splitting from Rose, I was entirely alone on Labor Day. I remember sitting quietly on my couch and noticing the experience of being alone. I wasn't lonely, just alone. An image of a hologram came to me, and I saw that all phases of my life are holographic, that space-time is interwoven past, present, and future. In the past, my life had been full. In the future, it would be full again. I would have a partner and lots to do on Labor Day, just not this particular one. I felt a great deal of peace with this realization.

I soon made a list of 20 qualities I wanted in my next partner. People sometimes ask if this is too mathematical, too clinical. For me, it was just the opposite. It was a form of surrender. I was setting the bar higher, clarifying to God/Goddess I was here for a higher purpose and I trusted that all my dreams would be fulfilled. I was clear that in my next relationship I was ready for a blissful connection on all levels — spiritual, intellectual, emotional, and sexual. I wrote that list, put it away, and enjoyed life as it unfolded.

Finally my dissertation was complete and I got the go-ahead from my inner guidance to start dating. I threw myself into the pleasure of meeting men who also wanted to meet me. I would sit at dinner across from a near stranger, only he didn't feel like a stranger. He was another being, a soul with a precious heart with whom I was blessed to spend time. We always had great conversations.

During this time, I experienced my first trip to India. As I was leaving the home of a new friend in Jaipur, my young hostess Shivani took both of my hands in her hands, looked deeply into my eyes, and said a prayer for me. I knew she was praying that I would find the right beloved when I returned to the United States. I don't remember putting out the "I want to find a husband" vibes to her, but somehow she knew.

In South India, I visited the shrine of The Mother, the spiritual companion of Sri Aurobindo, who had taken *mahasamadhi* (the death or passing of a saint) in 1973. Her devotees maintain her resting place with utmost tenderness and respect. Flower petals are freshly arranged daily in ornate patterns on her shrine. Devotees line up to file by the shrine silently, kneel briefly, then sit meditating in the surrounding courtyard.

I took my place in line. When it was my turn to kneel, I spontaneously placed my forehead on the marble, felt an immediate power rise up into my body and heard the words, "I will help you." Dazed, I stood up and moved on, but I carried with me a sense of presence, protection, and guidance.

The week I returned home from India, I received the news that I had been let go from a small part-time job. The person calling me was worried about how I would take the news, but I felt only gratitude and blessings. Something in me had shifted while in India, and I returned in a deep state of peace and trust.

An Ideal Partner

One month later, a man named Jim called me to go on a walk. I was excited. I had connected with him a year and a half earlier and had really liked him. I felt he would be a great match. But, at that time, he had been living with a partner, so I let any thought of dating him go completely.

On the walk, I soon learned that Jim and his partner had separated six months earlier. Two hours later, he learned that I was dating men, and our connection formed instantly. Tenderness and care welled up inside us, and our bond has been strong since that day.

It is hard to put into words how powerful my relationship with Jim was and remains. We have the most gutsy, passionate, grab-him-by-the-seat-of-the-pants-and-make-sure-he-knows-that-I-love-him relationship I've ever experienced. I can be more myself with Jim than I ever have with anyone — more smart, more silly, more creative, more joyful, more sexual, more non-sexual, more fierce, more soulful, more loving. This is what I had been longing for all along.

A week after our momentous walk, I sat him down in my living room and asked: *What are you most passionate about?* I was amazed as he opened a treatise on the technology he had developed for people with brain injuries. Here was someone who was as passionate about his creative work as I was! I have since realized that having a partner whose entrepreneurial spirit matches mine is an essential quality for a long-term relationship for me.

An amazing relationship is not necessarily perfect, and Jim and I do have our struggles. Interestingly, some of the things I wrote on my list of 20 ideal qualities turned out to be areas of difficulty. I wrote that I wanted a man who was spiritual rather than materially-oriented, saying it was okay if he didn't own his own home yet, as long as he believed that it would be possible one day.

Not surprisingly, we struggled financially as this had been an area of weakness for both of us. We then made a choice to heal our money karma. We began 12-Step work on debt, studied money sobriety, learned business skills, and read books like *The Four Steps to Financial Prosperity*. Within ten years and after much hard work and many divine blessings, our situation had completely reversed. I can vouch that financial sobriety works, and that it's possible to find financial peace and abundance.

I had also written on my list of 20 qualities that I wanted a man who didn't want children, or any *more* children. It turned out that a year after falling in love with Jim, I changed my mind and desperately wanted to have his baby! He had raised a daughter and was clear that phase of his life was over. I grieved that I had not met him at a younger age and that I was not the mother of his daughter.

Jim was open to hearing my grief and my desire. As an act of generosity and love, he joined me in exploring whether shared parenthood might be right for us, despite our precarious financial situation and our age. We considered creative options such as gathering a strong community of aunties and uncles — 6 of whom met with us to discuss their intended support — as well as fertility options such as donor eggs.

Ultimately, we stuck with the no baby plan. I now have a deep empathy for women who long to have a child and are not able to. I also strongly understand the benefits and freedoms of being childfree, as having children takes up enormous streams of energy in a woman's life.

I also now believe that many beautiful souls are looking to incarnate through good parents, and that we need to support the families around us. Those who parent are doing so on behalf of us all, on behalf of the evolution of our species, on behalf of our holographic selves who are those children they are raising.

Sex as a Healing Force

I feel deep satisfaction in knowing that I sought and found the life and partnership I always wanted. Being true to myself along the way, including sexually, made that possible. I held onto my desire and had the strength to release whatever wasn't truly fulfilling it.

In contrast to what I was taught as a child — that sexuality should be reserved for marriage — I have come to believe that sex can be a medicine to help us heal along the path, long before we meet an ideal partner. Good sex is like good meditation, good prayer or good yoga. It is a positive, evolutionary force.

I knew from the truth of my body that each particular connection was nourishing and healing; it was beneficial to both my partner and myself. I never doubted that. If I didn't feel that goodness, I didn't have sex with that person.

Healing sex has the quality of truth and power. Many times when I have an orgasm with Jim, I will feel the force of love moving through me, dissolving anything that is not of its essence, that is not pure love. Any worries or petty resentments are completely released. Sometimes I am brought to tears in this process. My best understanding is that the harmonious field of love energy between us is magnified in those moments, facilitating this release.

In my youth, my orgasms were more contained. As I have matured, I now feel the whole-body expression of the orgasm, and the integrated nature of the physical with the emotional and spiritual layers of my being. I feel every cell bathing in this blossoming energy.

Love has touched me deeply many times, supporting my emotional and spiritual development. Every encounter brought me closer to another human, another soul, who is ultimately a part of God/Goddess, a divine emanation. I can honestly say that I love all the emanations of the divine. And what an honor it is to be given the gift of a beloved.

About Laura J Cornell, PhD

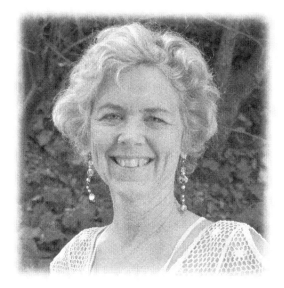

Laura J Cornell, PhD (*Yogeshwari*) is an award-winning speaker, author, sacred writing and sacred business mentor. She is Founder of Divine Feminine Yoga, through which she has directed eight online conferences empowering women through yoga, and where she offers coaching, retreats, online courses and leadership training for women worldwide.

Laura is author of the International Best-Selling book *Moon Salutations: Women's Journey Through Yoga to Healing, Power, and Peace*. In previous work as Founder of the Green Yoga Association, Laura spurred a national movement towards Green Yoga studios, produced two major conferences on yoga and ecology, and sold 10,000 non-toxic yoga mats through her living room. She has been featured in Yoga Journal, Yogi Times, L.A. Yoga, and Common Ground magazines.

www.DivineFeminineYoga.com
www.MoonSalutations.com

About Divine Feminine Yoga

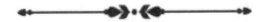

Divine Feminine Yoga was founded to help women heal ~ body, mind, and soul ~ so we can reach out to heal the planet. Join us to connect with like-minded women and to expand your voice in the world.

We offer:

- Global online conferences to inspire, uplift, and connect you with other lightworkers.

- Sacred writing circles, retreats, and mentoring.

- Sacred business courses, sister-mind support groups, and coaching.

- Yoga and meditation in beautiful Sedona, AZ.

- The opportunity to be featured in our books and online conferences.

Learn more and stay in touch:

DivineFeminineYoga.com
100 Sedona Street
Sedona, AZ 86351
888-423-8843

Also by Laura J Cornell, PhD

Moon Salutations:

Women's Journey Through Yoga to Healing, Power, and Peace

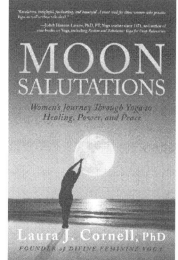

"Revelatory, insightful, fascinating, and beautiful. A must read for those women who practice yoga as well as those who don't." ~ *Judith Hanson Lasater, PhD, author* Restore and Rebalance

"Laura has given us a great gift through the birthing of Moon Salutations!" ~ *Nischala Joy Devi, author* The Secret Power of Yoga

"A wise, full moon of a book." *Amy Weintraub, author* Yoga for Depression

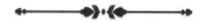

Available on Amazon and through Ingram Spark.

Claim your free Moon Salutations Audio with Mini-Posters:

MoonSalutations.com

Made in the USA
Columbia, SC
17 August 2021

43721213R00126